SEX PILLS

SEX PILLS

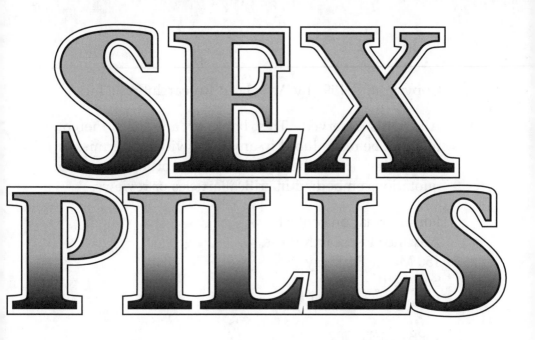

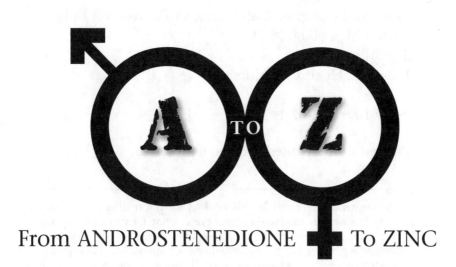

From ANDROSTENEDIONE To ZINC

What Works and What Doesn't

CARLON M. COLKER, M.D.

For information contact:
Advanced Research Press
150 Motor Parkway
Suite 210
Hauppauge, NY 11788

FIRST EDITION
Library of Congress Cataloging-in-Publication Data
Carlon M. Colker, M.D.
Sex Pills, A to Z
1. Sex   2. Health   3. Nutrition
1. Title
ISBN 1-889462-07-1

Printed in the United States of America

Published by: Advanced Research Press,Inc.
                         150 Motor Parkway
                         Suite 210
                         Hauppauge, NY 11788

Publisher/President: Steve Blechman

Managing Director   Roy Ulin

Art Director: Rob Wilner (DotCom)

Copy Editor: Carol Goldberg

Cover Design: Sam Powell (DotCom)

Photographs: Per Bernal

Models: Michael and Midajah O'Hearn

Printed by: DotCom

Sex Pills

DEDICATION

This book is dedicated to the entire staff at Peak Wellness for their tireless work in setting the highest of standards and leading the country in health and wellness.

TABLE OF CONTENTS

What Works and What Doesn't

ABOUT THE AUTHOR

Carlon M. Colker, M.D. is the Chief Executive officer and Medical Director of Peak Wellness of Greenwich, Connecticut (a center providing the full physician services of traditional allopathic medicine and preventive care along with the complimentary and integrative modalities of exercise therapy, therapeutic massage, and nutritional guidance). He has been in the health and fitness industry for nearly 20 years and to his credit, in the late 80's he helped design the first wellness program on the East coast. With a background as a former champion competitive bodybuilder and powerlifter, Dr. Colker is an internationally recognized consultant in health and fitness. He has worked with governments, large health systems, and private companies, as well as with Olympic and professional athletes and celebrities from around the world. He is a speaker for the American College of Sports Medicine, the National Strength and Conditioning Association, and the International Health, Racquet, and Sportsclub Association. In addition, he has a wealth of scientific research publications and articles to his credit. Dr. Colker is an attending physician at Beth Israel Medical Center in New York, as well as Greenwich Hospital, in Connecticut. As a special care physician, he takes care of the most critically ill patients in the intensive care unit at both St. Joseph Medical Center and Stanford Hospital in Connecticut.

Having appeared in such magazines as *Cosmopolitan, Runners World, Self, Glamour* and *Muscular Development,* just to name a few, Dr. Colker is a familiar and trusted person in the field of health and fitness. His commentary can be seen on national television as he is a regular guest on America's Health Network's "Ask the Doctor" segment and has appeared as a guest on such prominent shows as NBC's Health Segment. As one of the premier experts and speakers in health and fitness, Dr. Colker is often quoted in the media by such newspapers as The New York Times, Wall Street Journal, Seattle Times, and Boston Globe. He is a prolific writer with a host of feature articles and a vast readership to his credit.

Dr. Colker is also an established and successful general medical internist with a loyal patient following and, despite the rigors of his schedule, he makes ample time to care for his patients. He is active in public affairs and proudly committed to federal and local medical issues, having been appointed by the State of Connecticut to the honorable post of Assistant Medical Examiner and designated one of Connecticut's Probate Court physicians.

Sex Pills

INTRODUCTION

Sex—the primordial pleasure. The moment when all the basic needs of adequate nourishment, climate and cover are met, and a higher organism's natural homeostatic mechanism becomes even momentarily unchallenged, instinct turns quickly to procreation. Men and women are no different. The moment the need for survival and personal well being is no longer perceived as the primary focus, like any animal, we turn to sex. Perhaps therein lies the divine meaning of life—the purpose of which is to have sex. More accurately, the very purpose of life itself is to procreate. Life exists for no other reason than to simply perpetuate itself—too simple a concept for all the "great" philosophers and thinkers who have strived to identify a greater meaning or higher purpose. However, it is only the human who engages in the sexual act most of the time with no other purpose in mind except pleasure. Regardless of your belief system, be it religious in nature or politically driven, it is an undeniable truth that sex for pleasure far surpasses sex for procreation. In fact, I like to think humans are the only creatures who literally raise sex to nothing short of an art form.

As with any art or technology, it is a built-in natural tendency for man to want to improve upon it. It comes as no surprise then, that sex isn't any different. For eons man has wanted to make sex better, make it last longer, preserve sexual drive as one ages, reverse sexual dysfunction, restore a waning sex drive, and improve one's sexual prowess. To that end, man has engaged in a seemingly never-ending search for a magic pill or a potent elixir. This fixation is not with a mere few cultures, either. In fact, a healthy sexual preoccupation is a common denominator for every race of humanity if only looked at closely enough. Man has come up with products, injections, creams, gadgets, and contraptions, all with the intention of enhancing sex for pleasure in one way or another. Some are borrowed from nature, while others are synthesized in a laboratory.

Under the guise of "sex pills," the text that follows covers a plethora of substances and means intended to enhance sex. Some work, some don't. Some are brilliant in design and mechanism of action, while others are simply dangerous and stupid.

For the sake of easy reference, I have chosen an alphabetized method of presenting the information. Within this context, I have selected an approach that not only looks at the science behind a given product or means, but also examines the relevant anecdotal reports and conventional wisdom. In this way we safely avoid falling pray to ignorance and fairytales, while at the same time we avoid being blinded by science.

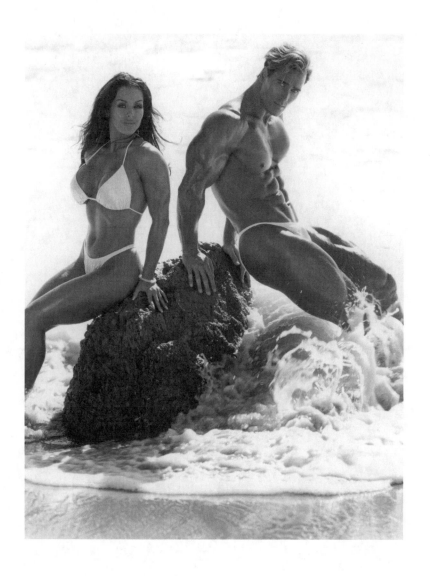

What Works and What Doesn't

(Evaluations of the effectiveness of herbs, drugs, nutritional supplements and other substances intended for sexual enhancement.)

Androstenedione

If the idea of taking a prescription medication as a sex pill is not appealing to you and you wish to take a natural route, you might consider *androstenedione.* Androstenedione is the direct precursor to *testosterone* (the male sex hormone known to enhance libido when in high concentration).

Most of the research supporting androstenedione alone as a substance that raises testosterone stems mainly from obscure foreign research articles, many of which date back to the 1960s. The primary marketing thrust stems from a notion that, in much the way dehydroepiandrosterone (DHEA) was advertised in the early 1990s, it serves as a building block for testosterone and therefore boosts levels in the body. While both hormones are in fact building blocks or precursors of testosterone, they differ in that DHEA is really the precursor to androstenedione, while it is androstenedione that is the direct precursor to testosterone.

A
B
C
D
E
F
G
H
I
J
K
L
M
N
O
P
QR
S
T
U
V
W
XYZ

FIGURE 1

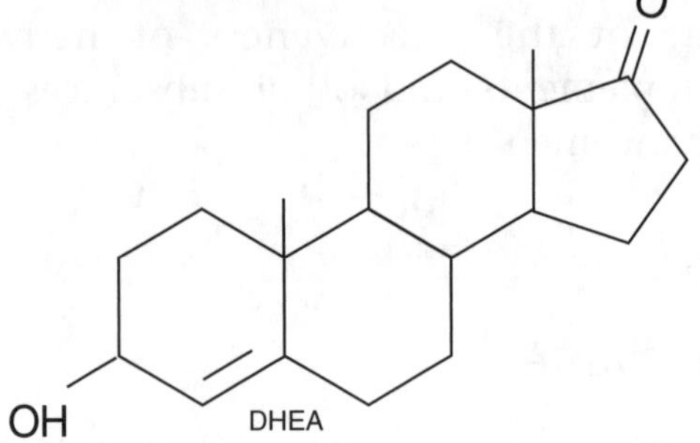

DHEA

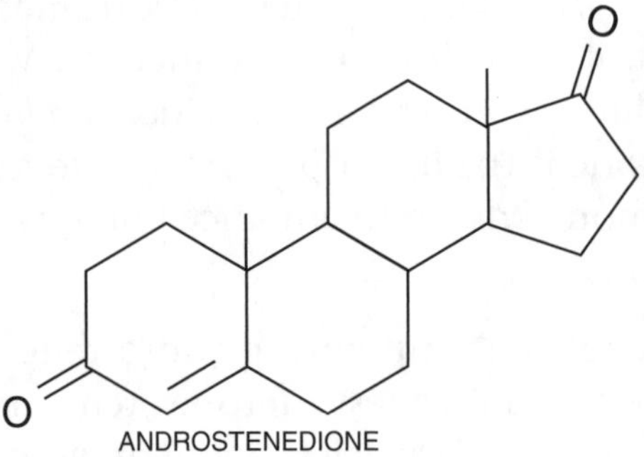

ANDROSTENEDIONE

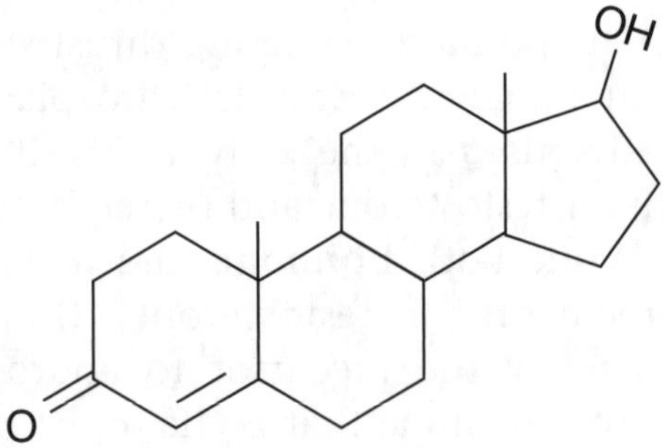

TESTOSTERONE

Keep in mind that this does not mean that androstene-dione is the "better" testosterone enhancer. Among many factors, the compound's "half-life" is a major consideration. The half-life of a substance is the amount of time it takes for the body to degrade it to half its concentration; the shorter the half-life, the less time it

Sex Pills

stays in the body. Compared to DHEA, androstenedione has an exponentially short half-life, thus hardly lending itself to a regimen of long-term use for the purpose of boosting testosterone levels. As such, to maintain significant levels in the body, it would have to be taken several times a day on a nearly continuous basis. In fact, it can produce a three-fold increase in testosterone within an hour or so, but after that, the concentration trails off exponentially.

Nonetheless, the logic for taking androstenedione over DHEA to enhance testosterone is that, because androstenedione is further along (or more terminal) on the pathway to the formation of testosterone, it is supposedly more likely to become testosterone in the body than DHEA. Added to that, DHEA taken by itself and not in the presence of an aromatase (estrogen) inhibitor, is a weak androgen (muscle builder) with only a minimal amount converted to testosterone in the male. It is only in the female that DHEA has been shown to produce a significant amount of testosterone.

Keep in mind that although androstenedione more closely resembles testosterone than does DHEA, androstenedione by itself is still not absolutely destined to become testosterone. In fact, androstenedione is also the direct precursor to estrone (an estrogen hormone). Thus, depending upon the physiologic milieu, androstenedione can quite easily become either hormone. As a matter of fact, in some settings, the conversion of androstenedione to estrogen can be more energetically favorable than the conversion to testosterone. In other words, there is no guarantee the androstenedione you take is going to become testosterone and not estrogen.

FIGURE 2

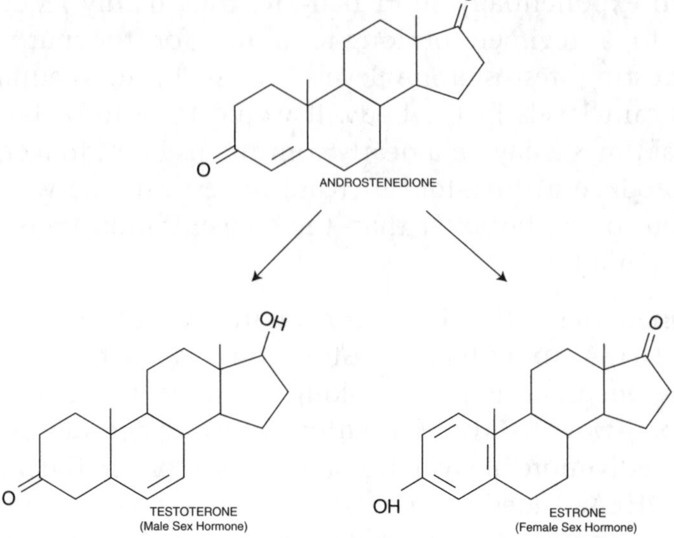

ANDROSTENEDIONE

TESTOTERONE
(Male Sex Hormone)

ESTRONE
(Female Sex Hormone)

In terms of chronic (long-term) use, there may even be an inherent danger for some people. Unlike a body that might need more estrogen (i.e., many post-menopausal females, total hysterectomy patients, or patients with some types of prostate cancer), in a body that does not warrant the estrogen therapeutically, there are a number of potentially deleterious side-effects that can accompany a high estrogen state. Such effects include menstrual disturbances, cancer, edema, gynecomastia, thrombocytopenia, as well as an association with disease states and illnesses like systemic lupus erythematosus (SLE) and thrombophlebitis.

Taking androstenedione on a long-term basis does not necessarily mean you will encounter one of these problems, but it is something to be aware of. In other words, if you take androstenedione for an extended period of time, you increase the chance that your system will

Sex Pills

convert it to estrogen in significant and potentially pathological amounts.

In addition, taking androstenedione by itself may be contraindicated in some people. For example, even if your body is free of disease but you are carrying a lot of fat on your frame, taking androstenedione alone for the purpose of boosting testosterone on a long-term basis would be ill advised. This is because conversion via aromatization (the process by which androstenedione becomes estrone) occurs to a significant degree in peripheral fatty tissue. This, in turn, opens the door to the estrogenic state and all the potential problems that go along with having too much of this hormone if your body doesn't need it.

As I see it, given the precarious and unsure destination of this hormone, taking androstenedione substance alone for a prolonged period of time is not advisable. Given that a long-term course of androstenedione for the purpose of anabolism via enhancing testosterone is indefinite, chancy, and possibly dangerous, one might ask what use, if any, does this substance have when taken alone? The answer to this is that on a short-term basis (although more research needs to be done), androstenedione alone may prove to be an excellent enhancer of male libido.

The key to enhancing your libido with this substance lies again in the assumption and the hope that the androstenedione you take is going to be converted into testosterone and not estrogen. Make no mistake about it. Just as it is foolish to take it long-term for the purpose of anabolism via conversion to testosterone, the odds of conversion to estrogen in short-term single dosing for the purpose of possibly stimulating libido are unfortunately no better.

However, the "advantage", if you will, of taking androstenedione in the short-term fashion is that, given the rapid pharmacokinetic metabolism of androstene-dione, even if it is aromatized to estrogen, you avoid long-term exposure to the estrogen formed. Thus, the chance that you would ever suffer any deleterious effects from the presence of excess estrogen would be unlikely.

With the assumption that the androstenedione you take is going to be converted to testosterone, we must also hope (for the purpose of libido enhancement) that the conversion occurs in an expedient manner. A delay in the short-term production of endogenous testosterone will do little in terms of your libido if timing is an issue. Unfortunately, you have no way of predicting or control-ling the rate of conversion (that's, of course, if you're lucky enough to convert in the first place). Nonetheless, anecdotal reports of androstenedione enhancing sex drive abound and are startling.

Regarding testosterone and libido, there is a paucity of information available. The fact is, the actual level of testosterone required for normal erectile function remains unknown. We do know there are "central" (located within the central nervous system) receptors for testosterone. These receptors act quite differently than those in the periphery, where a steroid hormone must go through the process of first binding to a target cell membrane receptor, then undergoing transport into the cell, binding to a cytoplasmic protein (also known in some scientific circles as a "heat shock protein"), forming a steroid protein-complex, and entering the nucleus of the cell, all to finally effect protein synthesis.

Thus, it is a fairly long process for a steroid to exert its effect peripherally (unlike a non-steroidal molecule like insulin, for example, which acts almost instantaneously in the periphery). In fact, as most anabolic steroid users well know, it can take weeks before any measurable action is seen. In keeping with this, it makes sense that the largely androgen-induced side effects also tend to occur with prolonged usage.

In contrast to this more peripheral phenomenon, there are many central receptors governed by a different and much faster mechanism of action. These central receptors are exquisitely sensitive to circulating hormone concentration (i.e., leutenizing hormone and testosterone). In the case of male libido, it is quite possible that small amounts of testosterone may temporarily give it a boost. Thus, with androstenedione producing a short-term increase or "spike" in serum testosterone lasting only an hour or so, it logically follows that it is a relatively safe and effective way of possibly eliciting a short-term and transient positive effect on male libido.

In addition, an important point to consider is that it is conceivable that androstenedione itself may exert a stimulatory effect on centrally located testosterone receptors. If true, this would eliminate the need for a lucky conversion of androstenedione to testosterone. Unfortunately, to date, there is absolutely no hard proof that these pharmacokinetics apply. Nonetheless, it suggests another mechanism to explain its speedy action and may also help account for the large number of people who unofficially report a positive influence on libido that seems to exceed a placebo effect.

In theory, if you take androstenedione infrequently in one-time dosing, you might experience a positive effect on libido while avoiding the possible untoward side effects of chronic androgen stimulation as a result of potential estrogen conversion. If we go on the assumption that the androstenedione you take will be converted to testosterone in a timely and expedient fashion, and that this testosterone (or possibly androstenedione itself) will exert a central effect to positively modulate libido, then we may have found a responsible, safe, and effective use for androstenedione.

Beyond simply "patch working" sexual dysfunction with a controlled substance, it seems as though androstenedione works by actually stimulating your libido. Given the rapid pharmacokinetic metabolism of androstenedione, the androstenedione you take can be quickly converted to testosterone. This quick single-step conversion is essential to reap the benefits of libido enhancement.

This particular mechanism of action of androstenedione relies heavily upon the transforming to testosterone. From here, testosterone acts on "central" receptors. These receptors act quite differently than those in the periphery, where a steroid hormone must go through a lengthy journey through cell membranes and ultimately into nuclear cytoplasm to exert an effect. Reflecting this mechanism of action, anabolic steroid users know it can take weeks before any measurable action is seen.

On the other hand, the central action of testosterone and libido enhancement relies on a central "neuro-hormonal" pathway that is governed by a different and much faster mechanism of action. These central receptors have been shown to be exquisitely sensitive to circulating hormone concentration, like testosterone and even leutenizing hormone. In the case of male libido, even a small surge in the blood concentration of testosterone stimulated by androstenedione may temporarily boost libido. With androstenedione producing a short-term increase or "spike" in serum testosterone lasting only an hour or so, it follows that it is a relatively safe and effective way of eliciting a short-term enhancement of male libido.

"Proposed Indirect Central Mechanism of Action of Androstenedione:"

Androstenedione (oral ingestion) ⟶ Testosterone (one step conversion) ⟶ Testosterone

Receptor (central stimulation) ⟶ Neuro Hormonal Response (activation of libido).

Interestingly, androstenedione may itself exert a stimulatory effect on the centrally located testosterone receptors I speak of. This mechanism of action is even faster than testosterone conversion because it alleviates a transformation step. This "direct" action of androstenedione on the central receptor provides yet another mechanistic explanation for the effectiveness purported by so many consumers.

"Proposed Direct Central Mechanism of Action of Androstenedione:"

Androstenedione (oral ingestion) ⟶

Testosterone (one step conversion) ⟶ Testosterone Receptor (central stimulation) ⟶

Neuro-Hormonal Response (activation of libido)

In my opinion, whether direct or indirect action, it is likely a combination of both pathways that explains why anecdotal reports of androstenedione enhancing sex drive abound. In either case, both pathways work toward the same result—enhancing your libido. Currently, from a non-prescription standpoint, androstenedione-based products effectively exert action by either quickly converting to testosterone or by acting directly upon central testosterone receptors to stimulate libido.

Interestingly, perhaps this mechanism of libido enhancement is also responsible for the large number of athletes from professional baseball, football, and basketball, down through the Olympic and amateur ranks that claim androstenedione improves their disposition toward competition. Many have claimed it improves their moods or gets them focused. Getting in the proper frame of mind, or getting "psyched up," for a competitive athletic event may not be all that different from tapping into one's libido. Perhaps there is some degree of crossover, and therein lies the key to understanding why so many athletes claim it helps them. Yet our knowledge of the pharmacokinetics of androstenedione simply doesn't support its use as a long-term testosterone enhancer. In much the same way one can use the theoretical short-term boost of testosterone from androstenedione to pepper one's libido, it follows that it would take no great leap of faith to accept the idea that androstenedione could very well augment athletic performance if taken prior to an athletic event.

Given this, the great fear for me as both a physician and a responsible clinician is that the so-called "pony-leaguer" or child athlete will get hold of this substance. The ramifications of oral ingestion of androstenedione can be devastating. The way a young body responds to the presence of a chemical substance, whether natural or synthetic, is far different than the physiological response of an adult. In particular, a child's body is exquisitely sensitive to steroid hormones in terms of both natural growth plate development and fusion as well as the cultivation and normal maturation of a proper endocrine and reproductive system. Simply stated, giving androstenedione to a child could be nothing short of horrific.

On the other hand, androstenedione for the adult male is currently accessible by the consumer and very affordable. One thing to keep in mind is that the dietary supplement industry is loosely regulated by the FDA so getting a high quality product is a serious issue. When

Sex Pills

buying androstenedione, stick with a trusted name brand in the supplement industry and don't waste your money with a mail order or no-name bargain brand.

Of further interest— if one accepts the premise that androstenedione positively modulates libido via its transient rapid conversion to testosterone and/or through a direct central action— is that if one's goal is to enhance libido as well as sexual performance, it makes perfect sense to consider combining two substances—androstenedione with yohimbine. The combination is sold in the form of a product called "AndroFuel,®" manufactured by TWINLAB® in Hauppauge, NY, and packs quite a wallop. Considering the synergistic benefits of this formulation, it would not be surprising to see this product popping (pun intended) off the shelves at healthfood stores across America.

The familiar substance yohimbine has an interesting mechanism of action which is discussed later in this text. It works extremely well when combined with androstene-dione to both stimulate desire and libido as well as enhance sexual performance. One can surmise that by combining both potential actions— stimulating libido via androstenedione along with staving off ejaculation via yohimbine— we may have finally arrived at the single most useful, safe, and effective natural formulation for both stimulating libido and enhancing sexual performance.

Angus castus

Angus castus is a homeopathic remedy popularized by the naturopathic physicians or "N.D.'s". Supposedly it helps with penile flaccidity and difficulty with male arousal. It is generally thought that this substance exerts its effect by blunting or countering the adrenergic or "sympathetic" response. This neuro-hormonal response is governed largely by what is called the "fight or flight" response. In other words, the system dominates when fear and anxiety are present. During such an episode, heart rate increases, pupils dilate, and often there is a sense of impending harm or even death that accompanies the situation.

Angus castus is also said to "warm" the penis, bringing in bloodflow that is essential for normal erection. Interestingly, practitioners claim that angus castus can help in all phases of male erectile dysfunction. Supposedly it can do everything from enhancing basic desire to improving erection.

Unfortunately, in spite of the proponents, the truth is that there is really no science to support the use of angus castus and few anecdotal reports.

Anti-estrogens

While the male sex hormone testosterone drives sexual aggression and prowess, the tempering force of the female sex hormone estrogen seems to do the opposite. Such is the balance of nature—men and women balance each other. Unfortunately, technology and the human condition have disturbed this balance.

Pollution of the air, water, and soil has disrupted nature's way. Chemicals and toxic elements like PCBs, DDT, dioxin, lead, mercury, and arsenic have poisoned our environment. Estrogenic medicines like birth control pills are wasted into our sewers or dumped into landfills, only to make their way back to our water supply for global ingestion.

Although these are facts, the theory is that this environmental molestation, caused by artificially introduced estrogens, can interfere with sexual development, hinder spermatogenesis and fertility, and impede sexual desire and function. It is a theory shared by many, and one that I am not quick to discard. It does not require a great leap of faith to imagine how such an effect could explain why the average sperm count has decreased by 40% since 1940.

Add to that hormonally manipulated livestock supplying our milk combined with the average low-fiber content in the American diet (low fiber lengthens the amount of time ingested toxic substances stay in the body and thus increases the absorption).

Indole-3-carbinole (I-3-C) is an enzyme-modulating agent found in cruciferous vegetables (i.e., broccoli and Brussels sprouts) and in fairly high concentration in cabbage juice; both are foods we don't eat enough of. This substance exerts an anti-estrogenic effect by diverting the conversion and production of a toxic form of estrogen to a less toxic form. This shift in estrogen metabolism has been demonstrated in cancer prevention research and holds a great deal of promise.

The primary problem with I-3-C is one of stability and shelf life. It seems that most raw material suppliers use desiccated broccoli to make pills instead of extracting I-3-C in its pure form. The reason is simple: price point. Expensive extraction technology for I-3-C at this time in response to the limited demand would translate to an unreasonable expense for the average consumer. Simply stated, I-3-C extracted in a concentrated and pure form that has a correspondingly stable shelf life would currently be far too expensive for widespread consumer consumption. So, until demand increases we cannot expect the quality of available and affordable I-3-C to catch up.

Another approach to counter excess systemic estrogen is to block its production from substances like androstenedione and testosterone, both of which can be converted to estrogen by way of "aromatization." In an effort to prevent aromatization to estrogen, some have suggested the use of aromatase inhibitors. The hope is to prevent the formation of estrogen and drive the reaction forming testosterone forward, as well as preventing any "end-point" conversion of testosterone itself into estrogen.

FIGURE 5

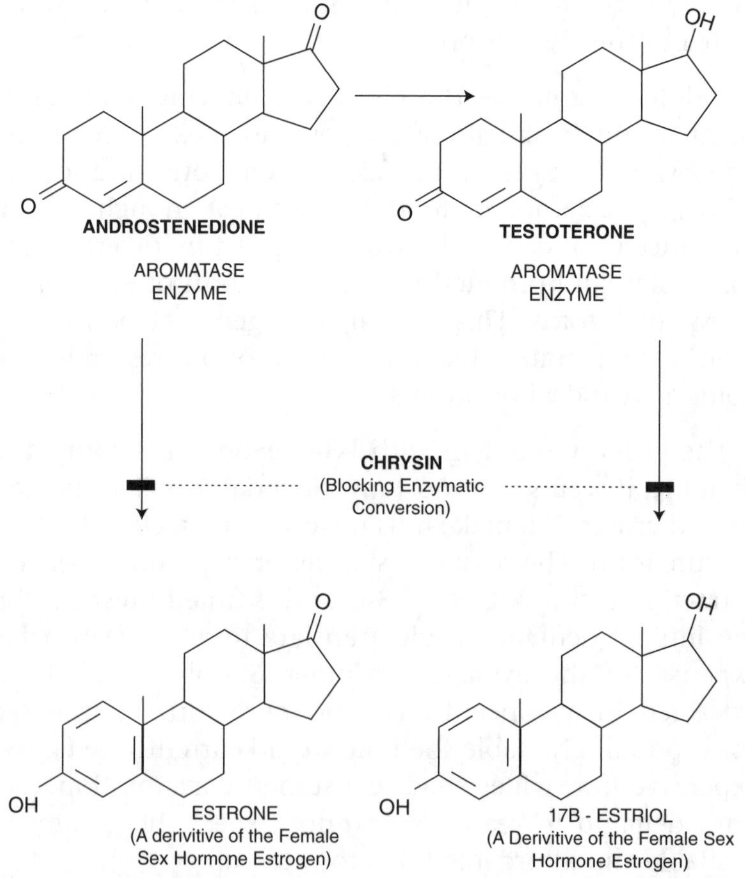

ANDROSTENEDIONE

AROMATASE ENZYME

TESTOTERONE

AROMATASE ENZYME

CHRYSIN
(Blocking Enzymatic Conversion)

ESTRONE
(A derivitive of the Female Sex Hormone Estrogen)

17B - ESTRIOL
(A Derivitive of the Female Sex Hormone Estrogen)

One such substance called "chrysin" (also known as flavone X) has been widely promoted as a compound to enhance testosterone formation. But, it suffices to say there has been a woeful and potentially dangerous distortion of the available research-based literature to support its use in humans for any purpose.

Chrysin was never tested in humans. Claims made for the purpose of marketing are based on a single in vitro study published in 1984. The study, by Kellis and Vickery, looked at aromatase inhibition by chrysin and other similar compounds. Although the substances tested successfully inhibited estrogen synthetase (also known as aromatase cytochrome P-450), the effect was seen in a bunch of human placental cells in a test tube! Hardly enough to draw "cause and effect" conclusions about the human body.

As a member of the family of "flavones", chrysin is among the higher order of natural plant substances known to inhibit aromatase and was, in fact, the most potent naturally occurring aromatase inhibitor of those tested by Kellis, et al. But don't be fooled by the term "natural," as there are plenty of substances in nature that aren't tested in humans because they can make you quite sick and even kill you. Chrysin may or may not be such a compound. While there are a number of bodybuilding products on the market that contain chrysin, the fact is we simply don't know what it can do. To date, there are no published studies showing that chrysin has any effect on aromatase in humans or any other living animal, including rats.

In terms of the future, it is quite possible that aromatase inhibitors may find a role in the treatment of some types of estrogen dependent cancers (i.e., namely breast cancer and metastatic disease of the prostate). Early studies have been done on cancer patients both in the U.S. and Great Britain, but further investigation is needed. In the meantime, the use of chrysin is growing in popularity within the bodybuilding community. So, with time we will find out one way or another whether it is as effective as some ergogenic gurus claim, or as toxic as some scientists suggest.

On the other hand, there are the "isoflavones" like soy. Although not an inhibitor of aromatase like flavones such as chrysin, soy is considered a weaker estrogen than estradiol and the other estrogen derivatives in the body. The result is that ingestion of these so-called "soy isoflavones" causes them to exert what we call a "relative" blocking effect on the effects of estrogen. Although soy does activate the estrogen receptor, it does so to a lesser extent than estradiol or any of the other estrogen derivitives.

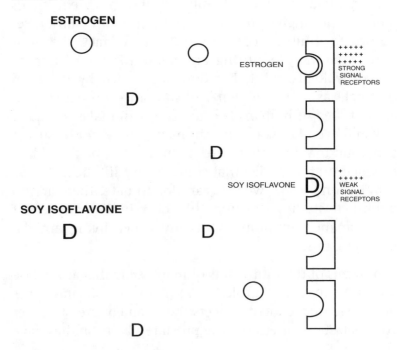

Soy is a common food substance well known to man, exhaustively tested, and most importantly, quite safe for almost everyone. Isoflavones and other naturally occurring flavonoids are present in the normal human diet in low but appreciable amounts (~1g/day). In fact, although this well understood mechanism does not actually block the formation of estrogen derivatives in the way a true aromatase inhibitor would, soy— by another mechanism not as yet understood— may be responsible for maintaining a low total serum estrogen. This may well explain the relationship between high concentrations of dietary isoflavones in the peripheral tissues and the relatively low plasma estrogen level we see in the vegetarian population.

Soy itself is a "phytoestrogen" and thus considered by some to be a reasonable estrogen substitute at some sites in the body or an alternative to hormone replacement therapy in the post-menopausal female. But understand that even though it is an estrogen analog, it is weak in its receptor activation when compared to pure estrogen. Thus, when competing for and occupying receptor sites (see figure 6) in a body that has an excess of estrogen, soy phytoestrogens will create a "blocking effect" simply by taking up space on the receptors yet not activating the receptor to the extent estrogen would.

Either way, given all of this, the hope of the anti-estrogen proponents is to suggest that they are effective sex pills in the adult male because they boost the production or increase the relative effectiveness of the body's testosterone. Unfortunately, despite all of the elaborate theories and the detailed mechanisms of action, none of these substances have yet to be shown to be effective testosterone ehnhancers. Thus, in terms of bolstering the libido, the likelihood is just as sketchy. Although many of these anti-estrogens have considerable

What Works and What Doesn't

medicinal promise and could prove quite effective as substances that prevent disease, it seems reasonable to concretely reject them as sex pills.

Antioxidants

The system of antioxidant free radical scavenging has received a great deal of attention in the area of disease control and prevention. Enzymatic, vitamin and mineral antioxidants play an essential role in nearly every bio-chemical reaction that occurs in the human body. These substances circulate throughout the system and literally pick up liberated harmful free radicals (molecules that have unpaired electrons that do damage in their search for "partner" electrons).

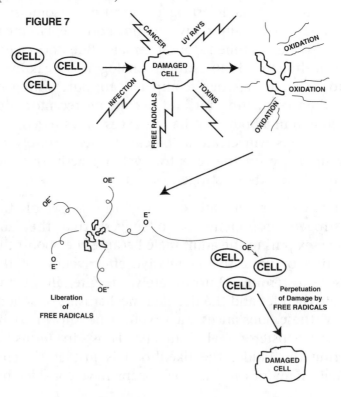

FIGURE 7

Scientists universally acknowledge the fact that free radical production through oxidation is constantly ongoing in our bodies. This process is an unavoidable consequence of cellular function. As cell lives turn over and new cells are produced, potentially dangerous free radicals are liberated. Thus, much of the research in nearly every discipline of science and medicine at one level or another has focused attention on cellular oxidation and the scavenging of free radicals at the molecular level. The antioxidant simply serves as an alternative oxidative substrate for free radical electrons, thus sparing otherwise healthy human cells from oxidative damage.

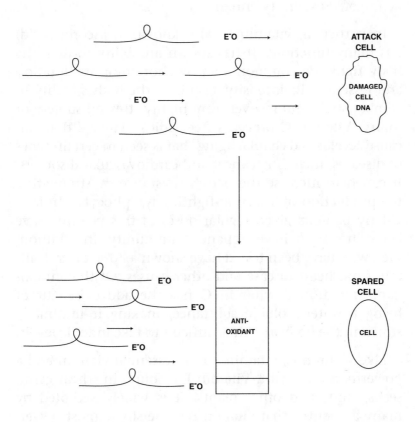

What Works and What Doesn't

Scientific investigators and health professionals generally recognize the role of free radicals in creating and perpetuating disease and illness. In fact, they are a common component of most of the chronic degenerative diseases, premature aging and premature death.

Interestingly, antioxidant substances like vitamin C, vitamin E, and the mineral selenium have all been widely recognized as powerful antioxidants with very real therapeutic value. Since the use of these substances has been so widely recommended for both general and specific ailments and purposes, it comes as no surprise that, right or wrong, somewhere along the line they would be targeted as virility enhancers.

In particular, vitamin C (also known as ascorbic acid) has many functions. It has shown an ability to help the body fight the common cold by shortening its duration and lessening its intensity. It aids in the body's ability to combat stress and recover from highly stressful surgery or injury. Vitamin C prevents free radical damage that can cause accelerated cellular aging that is seen in certain types of diseases, including cancer and cardiovascular disorders. It can help increase the body's resistance by stimulating the production of infection-fighting lymphocytes. In fact, elderly patients given regular doses of this vitamin have been shown to have enhanced immunity. In addition, men who have been tested have shown a 40% lower death rate from heart disease and other causes. Of the antioxidants mentioned, vitamin C has the added benefit of being a water- soluble substance, making it minimally stored in the body and thus difficult to take in toxic levels.

Like vitamin C, vitamin E is an essential vitamin and a powerful antioxidant. Vitamin E is found in wheat germ, seeds, nuts, and other plants. It is widely accepted by many a scientist that vitamin E is the single most powerful antioxidant in defending against harmful free radicals. Although it is a stronger antioxidant when compared to vitamin C, vitamin E is a fat-soluble vitamin and thus can also be stored in the body. This basically prevents safely taking "mega" doses. Nonetheless, as we age or become ill, the need for vitamin E increases.

Selenium is also an important antioxidant substance. Unlike vitamin C and vitamin E, selenium is a mineral. It is found only in plants and fruits that grow from the ground. Biologically, it has many functions. A major function of selenium is to act as a free radical scavenger, enhance vitamin E, and activate thyroid hormone. Selenium may also influence aspects of the immune system, reduce risks of cardiovascular diseases, and reduce risks of certain cancers.

In fact, a large-scale study at the University of Arizona demonstrated that selenium supplementation reduced the risks of breast, colon, prostate and lung cancers, while having no effect on cancers of the skin. Of interest is that there are many other diseases which suggest a role for selenium. Selenium in various test models has been shown to reduce the risk, effects and/or incidence of diabetes, arthritis, cystic fibrosis, malaria and sudden infant death syndrome, as well as HIV.

Selenium also activates the thyroid (a gland that regulates metabolism). We know that selenium deficiency can impair thyroid function and we know that excess body weight can lead to many diseases and complications. Therefore, selenium in essential to health and a vital life.

Despite the seemingly awesome power of these health-promoting agents, antioxidant substances can't really be considered sex pills. What we do know is that in animals moderate doses of vitamins C and E can enhance the ability of sperm to fertilize the egg. Unfortunately, at high levels, these elements can be toxic to sperm, interfering with sperm mobility and ultimately destroying them. In terms of selenium, studies have shown that this mineral is essential to the normal development of sperm. But beyond that, little is known.

As long as we are in the context of vitamins, although not really considered an antioxidant, vitamin A is occasionally touted as a sex pill. I should point out that although deficiency of vitamin A can cause impotence in some men, this should in no way imply that an excess will virilize a man or somehow enhance sex. In fact, an excess can be toxic.

In short, the antioxidant substances are perhaps best considered important for fertility and have little or nothing to do with sexual performance. The lack of science to support antioxidants as sex pills is mirrored by the paucity of anecdotal claims. Simply stated, if you're on a date and the man or woman you're with says vitamin C makes him/her better in bed don't get your hopes up for a very exciting night!

Apomorphine

Apomorphine is an oral agent for erectile dysfunction. It is a controlled substance that will only be available with a prescription, assuming it does come to market. Clinical trials are currently underway, but preliminary results are promising, revealing a 70% improvement in patients with psychogenic impotence. The mechanism of action centers around the ability of apomorphine to act as an opiate antagonist. Using this substance as a sex pill in otherwise normal physiology would constitute an "off label" use and something you would have to get your physician to agree to prior to trying. In fact, it is very possible it may not do anything in someone with a normal physiology.

Apomorphine is a pharmaceutical substance that is not likely without its side effects. Experimentation should be viewed with great caution, as any substance that exerts its action on the opiate receptor could have a multitude of systemic effects. Opiate receptors help to govern such sensory perception as pain, satiation, sleep/wake cycles, and certain levels of sensations of necessity and desire. Given the power of this system, it is easy to understand how one could become addicted to heroine or any other morphine derivative. Whether stimulating or blocking the opiate receptor, one should take such substances only if absolutely indicated and when the chance for possible benefits far outweighs the possible risks.

Argentum nitricum

Like *Angus castus, Argentum nitricum* is a homeopathic remedy distributed by naturaopathic doctors and seldom used by the general population. It is an herbal substance obtained by special order through alternative medical and naturapathic catalogues. Again, there is no scientific evidence supporting its use as a sexual enhancer for either men or women. In addition, given the relatively small numbers of people who have used argentum nitricum as a sexual aide, this hardly amounts to enough of a collective opinion to get a general consensus regarding its usefulness.

Even so, proponents claim that if erection fails on penetration, or if intercourse is limited secondary to unexplainable genital pain, argentum nitricum may help. According to the naturopathic physician, argentum nitricum helps best alleviate these complaints when they are accompanied by symptoms that worsen at night, with warmth, or when eating sweets.

Arginine

L-arginine is a naturally occurring amino acid. This substance is an oxidative precursor in the production of nitric oxide. Nitric oxide is necessary in low concentrations as an intercellular signal for penile erection.

"Normal Physiologic Mechanism Leading to Erection of the Penis:"

Parasympathetic Stimulation ⟶ Nitric Oxide Release ⟶

Guanylate Cylase Activation ⟶ Cyclic Guanosine Monophosphate

(cGMP) Production ⟶ Smooth Muscle Relaxation in the

Corpus Cavernosum ⟶ Increased Blood Flow to the Penis

It is surmised that under conditions in which nitric oxide is actively produced for a specific physiologic purpose, the concentration of L-arginine substrate from which it is formed can be a limiting factor. The faultiness in this logic is that the increased blood flow needed for erection results from low concentrations of nitric oxide, leading one to believe that it would be unlikely that low L-arginine concentration could be a limiting step, unless one was profoundly deficient in L-arginine substrate (a real "stretch", to say the least, in the American diet).

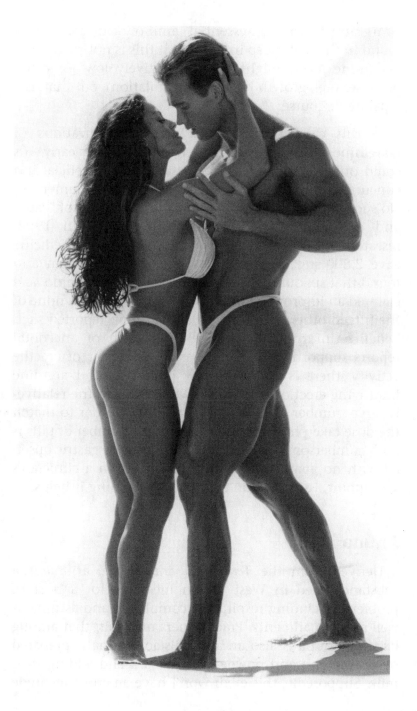

What Works and What Doesn't

Arginine is a non-essential amino acid commonly found in the diet. Keep in mind that this is not to say that L-arginine levels might not be relatively low for other purposes (i.e., growth hormone stimulation), but that, is a separate discourse.

In this case, the relative "high" concentrations of L-arginine given in a study performed in the early 90s could only be attributed as necessary and beneficial if a concurrent low serum L-arginine level was documented. No such measure took place, and thus, the issue of "cause and effect" comes to mind. Nonetheless, in 1992, researchers at New York University School of Medicine gave 2,800 mg of L-arginine to 20 impotent men and found that six out of fifteen men receiving the amino acid claimed an improved ability to get erections while none of the fifteen other men in the placebo group reported such benefit. Unfortunately, unlike the wealth of anecdotal reports supporting L-arginine as an enhancer of erectile activity, there is a true paucity of reports of L-arginine improving erections. This may well be due to the relatively large number of pills one must take in order to match the dose taken in the study. Such a high number of pills is both cumbersome, expensive, and may cause gastric upset, all with no guarantee of effectiveness. From a clinician's standpoint, I simply don't see people claiming it helps.

Arjuna

Derived from the *Terminalia arjuna* tree, arjuna is a substance used in West Indian medicine for a host of problems including respiratory complaints and asthma as well as heart ailments. Practitioners maintain that among its uses, arjuna is also an aphrodisiac. Arjuna is prepared by pulverizing and powdering the bark and adding it to milk. Supposedly, this elixir won't have an effect in single

Sex Pills

dosing. Instead, it is only after repeated daily administrations over a long period of time that arjuna exerts its sex-stimulating effect.

Active compounds have not been isolated to date and there exists no science to support its use. Given these facts (or lack thereof), it is my steadfast belief that one should never experiment with any substance distributors claim should be used over a long period of time even though little to nothing is known about its contents. This represents irresponsibility on the part of the dietary supplement industry. For safety's sake, such recommendations should be avoided at all cost. Simply stated, experimenting in one-time dosing of a substance is chancy enough, but chronic long-term use of a substance science knows little or nothing about is nothing less than scary foolishness.

Asafoetida

Yet another of the many substances from India purported to be an aphrodisiac, asafoetida is a Hindi spice from the *Ferula foetida* plant. Given its revolting taste, it comes as no surprise to me that it is also known as "devil's dung." But what does come as a surprise to me is that anyone would ever ingest such a repugnant substance without a certain guarantee of eternal ecstasy or at least gold at the end of the rainbow. Nonetheless, there are a few people who like it. But how this stuff makes it to the shelves of Indian grocery stores for mass sales, I'll never know.

Used as a treatment for various gastrointestinal complaints, asafoetida is believed to be an aphrodisiac. Simply stated, I can't see how this revolting brown material can be used for much of anything. If you're not used to it, you might find that the flavor alone could poison a rat. In short—I'd take a pass on the devil dung.

A B C D E F G H I J K L M N O P QR S T U V W XYZ

Ashwagandha

Here's another herbal "remedy" from India famed among practitioners as a substance that has been claimed to do everything from increasing potency, to enhancing libido, to even curing infertility. It is strange that when you push practitioners who use ashwagandha for specific answers as to what exactly it is best for and how it works, you tend to hear an earful in terms of all the things it supposedly can do while, when it comes to understanding how it works, you hear nothing but crickets.

The fact is, while small doses of ashwagandha probably won't harm you, its efficacy as a sex pill is merely of folklore. Without a stitch of scientific proof to support its use, or even significant reported anecdotal enthusiasm, doctors in India still dole it out to patients. With so many completely unconnected attributes apparently randomly connected to the use of this substance, it is no wonder many mainstream clinicians consider any positive results associated with the use of ashwagandha as only a placebo effect.

Asparagus

Is it any surprise that someone along the lineage of humanity took one look at this penis-shaped veggie and claimed it to be an aphrodisiac? Man (and I do mean man) has been fixated on the phallus since tribal times. In fact, entire cultures have been built around the human phallus as a centerpiece of worship. There is a strong and ancient perception that the human penis contains both the ability to produce the seed of life as well as unparalleled pleasure, and thus should be considered the center of being. Hence, it's not a shock that any innocent vegetable or fruit that even remotely resembles the human penis, would be subject to molestation by some society at one point or another throughout the history of mankind.

In this case, the lowly asparagus is our victim. Its use can be traced as far back as ancient Greek and Arab times when it was specially prepared for eating with spices and condiments so as to bring out the sex-enhancing properties of this phallic green.

Sorry, asparagus fans. The idea that the asparagus is some kind of aphrodisiac is based solely its shape and thus nothing beyond folklore. But, if after all I've said, you're still hooked on this "shape-function" notion, I at least suggest moving on to the banana.

Avena sativa

Derived from green oat straw (thus the saying "sowing your wild oats"), the botanical extract of *Avena sativa* has been identified as an aphrodisiac. Supposedly working by freeing up bound testosterone, avena sativa will, by way of testosterone, stimulate central receptors located in the brain that modulate sex drive.

Available in capsule form under the name "Vigorex", this sex pill is marketed to both men and women as a "super-potent aphrodisiac." But despite enthusiastic marketing claims, significant scientific research on avena sativa has yet to be accepted for publication in peer reviewed medical or science journals. This is not to say that research has not been performed. In fact, proponents are quick to point out a number of "in-house" studies and spurious case reports. Most of this information spawns from obscure "sexlogy" institutes at the periphery of mainstream medicine and science. Unfortunately, until these reports are accepted by legitimate medical or scientific journals, it is not possible to accept such observations as evidence supporting the use of avena sativa.

The next consideration is that of anecdotal reports. The so-called "word on the street" on avena sativa is that it is somewhat effective. Most "users" report a greater preoccupation with sexual thoughts and fantasies. They tend to spend more of their overall time fixated with sexual thoughts, acting out sexually with partners and indulging in masturbatory fantasies.

If you want to ignore the lack of legitimate published scientific support as it pertains to safety and efficacy, and go only on the anecdotal reports, there are a couple of issues you should be aware of. The first is that avena sativa seems to work better in men with low libido than it does for any purpose in women. The second, and perhaps more important issue, is my concern with an excess overall preoccupation with sexual thoughts. Afterall, while so many people want to "jazz up" their sex lives, I think far fewer want or need to have a perpetual pulsing signal in their heads telling them it's time for sex. Imagine trying to get a day's work in? So, while probably effective to some degree in solving a libido problem or two, based on its supposed mechanism of action in liberating more free testosterone, I wouldn't suggest taking it if you're a woman. On the other hand, men may very well benefit from this substance as we as scientists learn more about the way it works and the degree to which it is safe and effective.

Ayurveda

Ayurveda is a 6,000-year-old Indian method of alternative medicine that focuses on promoting health and longevity so that age-associated wisdom can be passed on through the generations. The key edict is one of structure and organization of daily life, concentrating on personal hygiene, work, food and nutrients, and proper sleep (no real surprises here yet). Coupled with these edicts is the harmonious use of herbal substances and extracts to assist in maintaining this inner balance.

The practice revolves around three governing principles in the body called "Vata", "Pitta", and "Kapha." In the simplest terms, when these principles and respective subdivisions are in balance, you have health. When they are not in balance, you have illness and disease.

A typical Ayurvedic treatment for sexual dysfunction might involve a mix of grape juice, onion juice, and honey to be taken at bedtime for 45 days. This will supposedly increase sexual energy and sperm count. Often, depending on your core Ayurvedic constitution, a practitioner may decide to add something called "trikatu" to your nocturnal swill. This Indian herbal preparation is a mix of ginger and Indian pepper. Bon appetite!

Note that there are quite a number of Ayurvedic treatments for sexual dysfunction and sexual enhancement. Amid this puzzling endless list, a few of the more common methods are listed separately in this text. All are as equally entertaining to read about as they are peculiar to contemplate taking.

Bios bande

From the *Roupala montana* tree found in throughout South America and the Caribbean Islands, a substance called bios bande can be extracted by soaking the bark in rum. Folklore has it that this bios bande (also known as macuocherie rum) has potent aphrodisiac qualities.

The bottom line here is that there is no science supporting its use and from the flimsy and fragmented anecdotal reports, I have every reason to believe that it is as much the rum content as it is anything else supporting its limited popularity. In fact, any sex pill or aphrodisiac substance with a bottom-line requirement to mix it with alcohol for the desired effect, can't really be seriously considered. Alcohol itself "disinhibits" an individual, which often leads to that person feeling a sense of sexual freedom and relaxation. This is frequently enough to stimulate the libido. Of course, in excess, alcohol will quickly squelch even the strongest urges.

Whether it is true or not that bios bande is an effective sex pill, or if it's just the booze at work, is a moot point since the paucity of supply makes this substance a veritable "rain forest delicacy" and pretty much precludes any practical use.

Bishop's Weed

Also known as ajwain, Bishop's Weed derives from a plant indigenous to India and some parts of the middle east. The seeds of the plant, known as *Trachyspermum ammi*, have been used for thousands of years by Ayurvedic practitioners in aphrodisiac food preparations. According to these practitioners, the substance enhances the ability of a man to have an erection and prevents premature ejaculation.

Sex Pills

Unfortunately, despite its long history, it has really never been scientifically tested and decisively analyzed. Interestingly, this substance seems to have a fairly specific role. Conversely, most substances in Ayurveda have such a multitude of effects that it often leaves one wondering if they really know exactly what a given substance specifically does. But this observation, when combined with the historic longevity Bishop's Weed has enjoyed, presents a curiosity to say the least. These are the hallmarks of a potentially efficacious and safe product that has not yet been proven. To be sure, we must wait for science to catch up.

Butea

This next non-descript moniker is derived from the name of the *Butea monosperma* tree in India. It is referred to by Indian natives as the "flame of the forest." It has made its way into Indian herbal medicine as a treatment for gastrointestinal upset and diarrhea, bleeding problems, and sexual disinterest. The leaves of this tree are said to contain its power. Unfortunately, these same leaves contain a chemical substance that can cause a precipitous fall in blood sugar and a racing of the heart rate that can be fatal.

My opinion? Until we know more scientifically, the only thing butea offers us is the "convenience" of being able to eat the potentially fatal leaves for an uncertain final lay, and still have the wood from the tree left over to burn for a cremation!

Cardamom

Cardamom, or *Elletaria cardamonum,* is an aromatic East Indian spice with seeds that are believed to contain a powerful sex drug. The seeds of cardamom are pulverized into a powder, then boiled with milk, and flavored with honey to make this sex elixir. Indian legend maintains that the spice can reverse impotence and stave off premature ejaculation.

A warning to the overzealous consumer is that an excess of cardamom is rumored to also cause the very things it is supposedly effective in treating—sexual dysfunction!

There is no science to back the claims from India and the only conventional wisdom that exists anecdotally seems to center around its use as a laxative. In fact, it is said that it is such a potent laxative that a frequent side effect is explosive, watery diarrhea (hardly the makings of a romantic evening).

Carnitine

Carnitine is a vitamin commonly seen on the supplement shelves and often pathetically misrepresented as a fat burner by overzealous marketers. The fact is, it is a substance essential for the metabolism of fatty acids (sorry to the ignorant—that simple fact alone is hardly enough to consider it a fat burner). A carnitine deficiency results in decreased energy. The utilization of carnitine to act on fatty acids in the production of energy occurs in the energy powerhouse of the human cell called the mitochondria. Any way you look at it, an excess of carnitine is not going to burn the flab off your hips.

At any rate, carnitine has been shown to be in unusually high concentration in an area of the testis called the epdidymis. This would lead one to believe that carnitine somehow plays an essential role in proper male reproductive function. Also of interest is that it has been shown that the higher the carnitine concentration, the more motile the sperm, while they become sluggish and developmentally stunted when carnitine is deficient.

The bottom-line on carnitine is that, although it could restore fertility in a man who might be carnitine-deficient, it is unlikely to be an effective sex pill for a man or woman. You're welcome to try it; it won't hurt you. But keep in mind that, as far as supplements go, carnitine is relatively expensive. When we start "talking dollars" you stand the chance of not only wasting your time, but your money as well.

Celery

Celery, the proverbial child's disappointment for a lunch-box health snack, somehow finds its way into the arena of sex pills. Tradition has it that the vegetable has some kind of sex-enhancing properties. Specifically the root or seed is believed to harbor its power. Further, legend has it that this portion of the vegetable should be served uncooked, as cooking or heating in any way is said to lessen its efficacy.

Subsequent to this, health food stores have distributed celery extracts for years to loyal consumers claiming a myriad of unrelated benefits in addition to its action as an aphrodisiac. Unfortunately, science gives absolutely no credence to their claims.

If appealing to your logical side won't work, try a little poetry. In this case, the truth about celery is probably limited to the Ogden Nash quote, "Celery raw develops the jaw, while celery stewed is more quietly chewed." You might also add the Colker adage, "Celery for lunch makes a healthy loud crunch, but as a sex pill, it won't give you a thrill."

Chasteberry

Chasteberry is also known by its scientific name of *"Vitex agnus castus."* Peripherally studied in the medical subspecialty of endocrinology, chasteberry has been shown to lower prolactin levels in women (a pituitary hormone that stimulates the secretion of breast milk which, when abnormally elevated, can cause a number of systemic problems). The production of prolactin in men in any appreciable amounts is abnormal and can lead to sexual dysfunction. Since it is a rare cause of sexual dysfunction in the male, the level of this hormone is seldom if ever checked. Thus, the theory is that there might be a population of men that have a "sub-clinical" abnormal elevation prolactin level that is impeding their sexual drive and function. This is not an entirely unreasonable theory, and fascinating to contemplate.

Well, if that condition isn't enough of a mouthful for you, chasteberry's research label name of "BP1095E1" should give you pause to think. Chasteberry is an interesting substance that might prove effective with more testing. But until then, I consider the mechanism of action in men to be a bit of a "mind bend" and applicable to only a sub-population. Regardless of its effectiveness in this sub-population, and even though this group may be larger than we had thought, it is still not widely applicable to the general population. And, if your physiology is normal and you suffer from no hormonal imbalance, it may do nothing at all for you. In short, the theoretical nature of its application coupled with the weak evidence of its efficacy to date is only matched by its poor availability.

Chocolate

Derived from the beans of the cacao tree, also known as *Theobroma,* chocolate has a long history of being viewed as an aphrodisiac. As early as ancient Aztec times, king Montezuma supposedly consumed massive amounts of a cocoa drink on a daily basis prior to entering his harem with the belief that it was an aphrodisiac. This "food for the Gods" was not limited to the Aztecs. In fact, the ancient Mayan civilization also valued chocolate to the point that only the upper class elite and greatest warriors were permitted the enjoyment of chocolate consumption.

By the 16th century the Spanish Conquistador Don Cortes brought chocolate back to Spain from Central America. Shortly thereafter, the Catholic Church determined chocolate to be an evil vice and the drink of sorcerers. Fortunately, by the 17th century, the Swiss began toying with chocolate, sweetened it, and invented a process called "conching" in which chocolate takes on a velvety and creamy consistency. That was all that was necessary for the chocolate craze to begin and for its popularity to sweep across Europe, gaining monstrous momentum with each passing year.

Nonetheless, chocolate remained a food for the rich primarily as a result of the heavy import duties. Such expense was passed on to the consumer, making chocolate a bona fide luxury well into the 19th century. In fact, it wasn't until 1853 that the exorbitant duties were reduced and the pleasure of chocolate reached a broad-based population.

In terms of chocolate as an aphrodisiac, there have in fact been some interesting compounds isolated from chocolate that may contribute to its reputation. The first, phenylethylamine, is a substance that exerts a psycho-stimulation of the brain akin to that of amphetamines. Theobromine, also a chocolate constituent, can act as an antidepressant and is said to mildly stimulate the nervous system. The caffeine found in chocolate can stimulate wakefulness and decrease feelings of fatigue. Seratonin, a potent neurotransmitter in the brain, regulates much of our perceptions about our environment including but not limited to excitation and our sleep-wake cycle. Lastly, let's not forget good old sugar as an important ingredient in "jump starting" a sluggish metabolism. Chocolate is high in this cane derivative and is likely responsible for much of the reported euphoric effects.

Unfortunately, Hershey lovers of the world, despite the wonderful virtues of these individual components and apart from sugar, chocolate itself has a relatively low amount of the substances mentioned. In fact, in order to take in clinically significant amounts of these chemicals with chocolate as the source, the average-size man or woman would literally have to devour pounds of the stuff. The result of which would leave you so fat that I question whether you would feel very sexy at all. But hey, it seemed to work for old Montezuma. Of course, those were "special" times of powerful motivaters such as human sacrifice and the like.

Chuchuwasi

A member of the *Genusm maytenus,* chuchuwasi is a tree bark preparation native to Peru and Columbia. The Peruvian Shphibo tribe prepares the bark for oral liquid ingestion by soaking it in cane liquor, while the Siona indians of Columbia simply soak the bark in river water to make their elixir.

Either way, since ancient tribal times, chuchuwasi been used as an aphrodisiac, as well as a potent muscle relaxant and treatment for joint pain and rheumatism.

Apart from South-American folklore, there is little information to support its use as a sexual aide. Nonetheless, the popular nature of this substance and significant anecdotal reports of efficacy have stimulated enough interest in chuchuwasi for it to be at least superficially studied. Interestingly, unlike many esoteric aphrodisiac substances, the active constituents of chuchuwasi have been isolated and are currently being tested. It may hold promise for the future as a sex pill of some kind but we are probably years away from knowing for certain.

Cinnamon

Also known by its scientific name *Cinnamonum camphora,* cinnamon has long been used as a popular spice and medicinal herb. Leaves and roots are crushed into a powder that, although quite flavorful, has no known action as an aphrodisiac. Despite the fact that only a few historic misguided souls claimed it made an effective sex pill, I am forced to wonder why it keeps resurfacing in non-scientific literature.

The truth is that active compounds of everything from camphor oil, to cineol, to fatty acids, to mannitol, to safrole, have all been isolated from cinnamon. An excess amount of cinnamon is said to block the absorption of iron and other vital minerals. Also, these isolated substances in significant amount can act as anything from a potent diuretic to a lethal carcinogen. Worse yet, in mega-doses, cinnamon is said to cause dizziness, convulsions, and even coma (although I never heard of any such case).

Science still gives it some attention. A fairly recent study, although quite peripheral and poorly designed, cited cinnamon as a possible aromatic aphrodisiac (i.e., by smell only). The take-home message here is that you might decide to sprinkle a little here or there for flavoring, and that's okay. Just be sure you stop short of crediting this spice with powers it simply doesn't have.

Cloves

Dried cloves are from the flower of *Jambosa caryophyllus* and are referred to as an aphrodisiac in ancient Chinese and 17th century Swedish literature. Legend has it that when consumed as a drink, it will restore and even enhance a man's sexual desire.

Although modern chemistry has isolated active compounds from clove, including eugenol, vanillin, and amyl ketone, they seem to contribute more to the powerful aroma and taste than to any element of sex drive.

My feelings here are simple. Tasty spice, lousy sex pill.

Cotton

Amazingly, in some regions of Africa, India and Pakistan, the cotton plant has been traditionally considered an aphrodisiac. Also known by its scientific name *Gossypium herbaceum,* the root and bark portions are believed to be sex stimulators.

Although never proven scientifically, there is strong cross-cultural evidence that cotton exerts a potent effect on both the female and male reproductive systems. The substance seems to be able to manipulate menstrual flow in the female and block sperm production in the male. Whether or not that means that cotton could be a potential abortifacient or male contraceptive remains to be seen. Either way, it certainly is doing something. But, until research proves otherwise, I strongly advise steering clear of a substance with such powerful but as yet ill-defined systemic effects.

Damiana

Damiana (also known by its scientific name *Turnera diffusa)* is a medicinal shrub found in the Mexican Gulf. It has been used since the late 1800s as an aphrodisiac and sexual ability enhancer. We know that damiana can stimulate muscular contraction of the gastrointestinal tract, but it can also seriously interfere with the absorption of iron and other minerals when taken internally.

As legend has it, this bitter-tasting herb is supposedly a "divine gift" with the power to rejuvenate the sexual prowess of the aging and restore youthful virility. Unfortunately, there is not a single stitch of scientific evidence, study or otherwise, to support its efficacy. Equally disappointing are the relatively small numbers

A
B
C
D
E
F
G
H
I
J
K
L
M
N
O
P
QR
S
T
U
V
W
XYZ

What Works and What Doesn't

59

attesting to its effectiveness. It seems that high honor and praise for this treatment comes mainly from the alternative practitioners that recommend it. These practitioners use it as a mild diuretic and prescribe it for urinary tract infection. History also holds that it was used as a cure for infertility. Seldom ingested alone or in raw or pill form, damiana leaves are traditionally sun-dried and prepared as a tea mixed with other herbs.

Similar to Spanish fly, its mechanism of action appears to center around its ability to induce a mucosal irritation and flushing. In particular, it irritates the distal urethra at the head of the penis. Supposedly, this irritation makes the user exquisitely sensitive to touch stimulation— ouch! Not my "cup of tea," if you ask me.

Datura stramonium

Like mandrake (discussed later in the text), datura stramonium is a member of the potato family. Reportedly, it was used in Europe centuries ago as an aphrodisiac. Also known as thorn-apple, *Datura stramonium* is literally deadly. In fact, it is such a toxic poison that even the most minuscule of doses can kill a man.

It always amazes me how substances like this are ever popularized as aphrodisiacs, or anything else for that matter. Perhaps the fixation with death spoke for its potency. Maybe just the thought that such a substance could so easily kill was some kind of peculiar "turn-on" in the Old World. Either way, how the lore of such a substance survives the ages is perhaps even more perplexing to me. It's disturbing, yet fascinating, to think about this dark corner of the human psyche.

Dehydroepiandrosterone (DHEA)

Dehydroepiandrosterone (DHEA) is a steroid hormone secreted by the adrenal glands. It is the direct precursor to androstenedione, which in turn can become either testosterone or estrogen (see figures 1 and 2). DHEA levels are relatively high at birth, rapidly taper in childhood, rise dramatically during puberty and throughout young adulthood, and begin to plunge during old age. Interestingly, only humans and apes share this unique and perplexing cycle.

DHEA also exists in a "sulfate" form called dehydroepiandrosterone (DHEAS). Produced and secreted exclusively by the adrenal cortex, DHEAS is the most abundant steroid in human serum. Despite its commonplace nature, like DHEA, DHEAS is equally mysterious in terms of its exact purpose.

DHEA does seems to hold promise in the area of the collagen vascular disease systemic lupus erythematosus (SLE). According to several California researchers, it seems SLE patients taking DHEA require less prednisone to manage their illness. According to recent research and ongoing preliminary studies, DHEA may also be useful in staving off or preventing osteoporosis. Anecdotally speaking, DHEA has been reported by a fairly significant number of individuals to make them simply feel better. My own limited clinical experience with DHEA, and that of my colleagues, seems to lend a thin arm of support to the ability of DHEA to bolster a subjective sense of wellness in males over the age of 40.

But there is simply nothing in the literature of any significance to warrant even considering DHEA by itself as a sex pill. It neither enhances drive or libido, nor does it contribute to performance.

DHEA appears to be less problematic in male consumption than in female consumption. One suggested application is that it may be best used combined with a substance like saw palmetto in a health maintenance formula for older males.

Dong quai

Simply stated, dong quai is probably the most widely used herb among Chinese medical healers. They seem to put it in just about everything from varicose vein formulas to heart elixirs. The theory is that it works by promoting healthy circulation around the body. In fact, many commercial sex pill concoctions slip this substance into their mixes with the hope that it will help deliver more blood to the genitals by opening constricted blood vessels. Of added interest is that, for whatever reason, its use is generally considered to be more effective for women than men. In fact, some more traditional practitioners caution against giving it to men at all.

Don't count on science to support this one as a sex pill. There is no reliable scientific indication that dong quai is either safe or effective. Anecdotally, on the other hand, reported usage abounds. But don't spring off your coach and race to Chinatown just yet—reviews as a sex pill are shaky and mixed at best.

Eleutherococus senticosus

Used by practitioners of Traditional Chinese Medicine (TCM), *Eleutherococus senticosus* is a naturally occurring herbal substance prescribed for disorders of the genitourinary tract. It is often combined with acupuncture for supposed greater systemic effect.

Eleutherococus senticosus is considered by most TCM practitioners to be a very effective treatment of impotence. Although apparently similar to ginseng, *Eleutherococus senticosus* has an advantage in that it does not exert an untoward effect on the kidneys (TCM practitioners claim that Panax ginseng taken in excess over time burns out the kidneys).

The mechanism of action is believed to center around the ability of *Eleutherococus senticosus* to increase the flow of blood in the genital area. However it works, eleutherococus senticosus actually seems to have some merit as a treatment for impotence. However, calling it a sex pill is another story. It could quite possibly enhance normal sexual activity but I know of no TCM practitioner that would prescribe it for these "recreational" purposes. Of course, as with other TCM products, both availability and cost can factor in to dissuade even the most motivated consumer.

Equisetum arvense

Considered a type of horsetail, *Equisetum arvense* is a plant preparation used by Swedish herbalists as a sexual enhancer. It is believed to reverse impotence and strengthen libido. As with all forms of horsetail, its active component is believed to be silicon. The problem here is that by itself silicon has never been shown to be effective from a medicinal standpoint. It may well be that there is another active component not yet identified, but that is of course only if you are convinced that *Equisetum arvense* works in the first place. I, for one, without either science support or significant anecdotal claims, am far from certain.

Fennel

Fennel, also known by its scientific name of *Foeniculum vulgare,* dates back to ancient Egypt where it was used for a variety of medicinal purposes. However, it was not until ancient Greece that healers discovered its use and popularized the widely held belief at the time that fennel had sex-stimulating properties. That simple label put on it by the Greeks allowed the reputation of fennel to take on literally mythical proportions and thus disseminate down through the ages. History has it that fennel was an integral part of festivities and often the focus of celebration. As the Greeks adorned their bodies with the leaves of the plant, ingestion of the fennel seeds supposedly propelled them into a sexual frenzy. (Sounds more like a Roman orgy to me).

Interestingly, these were not the only ancient cultures to celebrate the virtues of the fennel seed. In fact, fennel fixation spans many a culture and is found in ancient Hindu scripture as a prescription for sexual rejuvenation.

There is virtually no science to support fennel as a sex pill, however. Its chemical constituents have been isolated and studied, revealing no substance usable as an enhancer of sex. Nonetheless, the reputation of fennel is multicultural and universally legendary. This might lead one to believe that perhaps fennel contains a substance within it that has not yet been identified as an active molecule. This wouldn't be the first time folklore became fact. Only time and science will tell us for sure.

Fenugreek

Derived from the plant trigonella *Foenum-graecum,* fenugreek is one of the most ancient of Chinese botanical remedies. The pods of this plant are harvested, cleaned, and roasted for medicinal purposes and for use in cooking. It is a widely held belief that various isolated constituent chemical compounds act as sex hormone precursors in the body. Thus they exert a libido-enhancing effect that is supposedly equally effective in both men and women.

As legend has it, fenugreek's potency as a sexual enhancer and cure for impotence centers around the fact that portions of the plant itself actually resemble a goat's antlers (I hope you're sitting down for the rest of this). Consistent with the beliefs of numerous ancient cultures, when the male phallus is structurally demonstrated in nature, it quite often follows that its ingestion is believed to endow the consumer with sexual prowess. Need I explain more? I put these types of assumptions right alongside things like the ancient ritual from Central America of eating the heart of a warrior you defeat in battle in order to inherit his power. Although not quite as gruesome, the notion of consuming fenugreek with the idea that it is some kind of sex pill is just as "loopy."

Flower Remedies

Legend has it that, when sexual dysfunction has an emotional cause, flowers may be the answer. Homeopaths and herbal specialists suggest pink monkey flower if low self-esteem, poor self-confidence, and sexual insecurity pervade. If anxiety stemming from a fear of a repeat performance of a previously disappointing episode of impotence is the limiting factor, "experts" say sticky monkey flower (no kidding, that's the name) may be the answer. Additionally, if impotence is caused by trauma or other physically-induced cause, Star-of-Bethlehem may help, according to these self-proclaimed experts.

But sarcasm aside for a moment, the problem I have with these remedies is that, in my experience, they fail to be supported by both science and anecdotal reports. Simply stated, these substances have been taken by only a relatively small number of people. So, how one claims to be an expert when neither science nor conventional wisdom can back up what he or she offers is a mystery to me. But this should in no way imply that it is impossible for these or any other substances to be effective. It just makes it extremely unlikely. One must keep an open mind. For now, consider flower remedies fairly harmless tertiary options at best.

Garlic

Garlic, or *Allium sativum,* has been used since Egyptian times for just about everything from infectious diseases to mood problems. Most students are familiar with the legends of great Olympians using garlic before feats of strength. So it should come as no surprise that somewhere along the line the association was made between the power of enhanced sexual relations and the ingestion of garlic.

As an aside, recently there has been a great deal of talk about garlic as a treatment for elevated cholesterol. Unfortunately, more recent studies simply haven't strongly supported its use for this purpose. On the upside, garlic contains a plethora of vitamins and mineral substances as well as an amino acid called "allin" and its related powerful antioxidant compound "allicin".

However, despite being a delicious addition to dinner cooking and simply an overall healthy food, there is currently no scientific evidence indicating that garlic is in any way a sexual enhancer, nor are there appreciable anecdotal reports supporting its use.

One simple caveat, though. If you do decide to try it and it works for you, check out your partner's reaction to your breath and remember that it's unlikely he or she will be as "turned-on" as you if they haven't also had garlic!

Ginger

Also known as *Zingiber officinale*, the medicinal applications of ginger abound primarily throughout Asian history. This herb can either be ingested whole, prepared with food, or actually ground into a sticky paste and rubbed on the body. The latter is perhaps the most bizarre, as ancient texts describe not only rubbing ginger paste on the abdomen, but also on the genitals and anus to exert its desired effect. This effect is described as curing impotence in men and creating uncontrollable desire in women.

Forget finding science to support these claims because there is none. This use of ginger as a sex pill is pure fairytale and is not even well supported by anecdotal claims. In fact, the only medicinal purpose which the anecdotal reports seem to reasonably support is the use of ginger as a weak to moderate treatment for nausea and motion sickness. Other than its possibility as a substance that might settle the stomach, ginger is best left as a great flavoring agent.

Ginkgo biloba

From the ginkgo tree, ginkgo biloba is truly a fascinating substance. The fact is, even its origin is unusual. The ginkgo tree, also known as the maidenhair tree, is considered a "living fossil" because it is the only surviving member of the 200-million year old *Ginkgoaceae* family, thus making it the oldest living species of tree on earth. Perhaps one reason for its mysterious medicinal properties is that it is remarkably resistant to disease and pollution. This fact perhaps best accounts for its resilience and incredible longevity. Some trees are believed to be literally thousands of years old. You should check out Central Park in New York City where ginkgo trees abound as a successful import.

The leaves of these ancient ginkgo trees have been used in Chinese herbal medicine for more than 5,000 years. Thus, as is true for ginseng, when it comes to ginkgo biloba I am hesitant to quickly discard or refute claims about a substance that has stood the test of millenniums of time.

In fact, the relatively conservative mainstream scientific community seems to have taken on an interest in this rather unique substance. In the last decade, hundreds of scientific papers have been published detailing human experiments using ginkgo. The greatest emphasis here seems to be on the power of ginkgo as an antioxidant with the specific ability to open up terminal blood vessels and thus power circulation. If this mechanism of action is true, then it would perhaps explain why some extol its virtue as a sexual enhancer.

Of particular interest is a specific extract of ginkgo called "EGb 761" or simply "EgB" for short. It has been used for years in Europe to alleviate the symptoms associated with numerous cognitive disorders (i.e., dementia). Subsequently, perhaps the best known study to date on ginkgo was completed and accepted for publication in the prestigious *Journal of the American Medical Association* in 1997. The study looked at the safety and efficacy of EGb in Alzheimer's disease and multi-infarct dementia. It lasted 52 weeks and involved 309 subjects.

Much to the chagrin of many of my more conservative colleagues that *JAMA* would even entertain publishing such "herbology", EGb proved to be not only safe but effective in stabilizing and improving performance and functioning in demented patients over six months to a year.

One caveat to keep in mind with regard to ginkgo is that it should not be combined with aspirin. This unfavorable combination may result in multi-organ system complications of an as yet unclear degree of severity. This untoward effect is currently being investigated. Nevertheless, if the combination is avoided and daily dosing is less than 240 mg, it seems to be safe.

The question really then becomes one of examining its efficacy as a sexual aide. In keeping with the effect of ginkgo on the cognitively impaired and the supporting anecdotal claims that ginkgo is a sexual enhancer, the

explanation may have as much or more to do with its ability to sharpen the senses than with improving blood flow.

Perception and sensation are essential in all stages of sex whether general interest/libido, arousal/excitation, or performance. When perceptions are dulled, interest in sex naturally wanes. The most common reason in our society today is fatigue. Plain and simple, people today are overworked and stressed. They return home exhausted and out of gas. It can be understandably difficult to realistically expect a spouse to be interested in sex after a stressful day when he or she simply wants to eat, watch television and fall asleep. In practical and theoretical terms, because it heightens one's senses, it is easy to see why so many seem to respond favorably to the use of ginkgo. If that's your problem, give it some consideration. It may be worth a try.

Ginseng

Ginseng is a root commonly used in China, Korea, and India in raw form and as tea. As a food, spice, condiment and cure-all, it has been considered by these cultures over thousands of years to have powerful medicinal qualities. Among the wide range of traditional uses, the most common benefit attributed to this root is the enhancement of sexual function, particularly in men.

One proposed theory about the mechanism of action of ginseng is based in its active compound ginsenoside. Researchers believe ginseng improves sexual function by increasing hormone levels. Supposedly, this is accomplished by stimulating the body to produce more testosterone. Supporting this notion, ginseng has been loosely shown to increase sperm production.

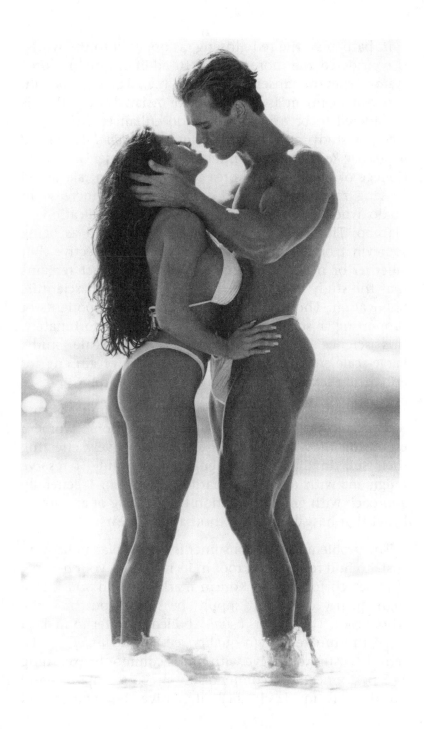

What Works and What Doesn't

71

In particular, the red ginseng, as opposed to the white, is considered the more potent. In addition, of the three major types of ginseng available (i.e., Panax, Siberian, and American), it is the Panax or Asian variety that is considered to be a powerful libido enhancer. In fact, in 1995, a study published in the *International Journal of Impotency Research* and conducted at the Yonsei University College of Medicine in Korea found that men taking red ginseng reported increased activity and an increase in libido when compared to antidepressant medication or placebo. This study has been largely criticized as being somewhat biased from a socio-dynamic perspective. But whether or not you believe the critics, the fact remains that the study was accepted in a peer-reviewed scientific publication. Therefore, one cannot accuse proponents of supporting a substance without science. Unfortunately, this science is based on only a small-scale study. Large-scale studies examining the efficacy of ginseng for enhancing sexual function have yet to be done.

Anecdotally, I have heard a tremendous number of case reports, mostly from men, but also from some women, espousing the virtues of ginseng on positively effecting their sex drive. Until further scientific study, I reserve judgment with a sort of guarded optimism; I generally approach with great trepidation the refuting of an idea or belief that has survived for thousands of years.

The problem for the consumer is one of availability and cost. To find red ginseng root in its raw form, your best bet is to search for a good Korean market. When you find a high quality consistent supply, be sure to purchase the whole root. This root is usually boiled in water to make a tea. Unfortunately, high quality red *Panax ginseng* can be terribly cost- prohibitive with prices commonly exceeding $45 per ounce. The commercially prepared capsules and powders are much cheaper alternatives but you should only use market name brands. Inferior products should not be considered, as the concentration of active ingredients in some of the "no-name" brands I've seen is nothing short of abysmal.

Like any substance, one thing to keep in mind when using ginseng as a sexual enhancer is not to overdo it. Here is a rare case where science does not seem to show any untoward effects from taking ginseng, yet the wisdom of Traditional Chinese Medicine (TCM) practitioners tells us otherwise. It seems these practitioners believe that using an excess of Panax ginseng can tax the kidney. Remember, this adverse effect has never been demonstrated in the scientific literature, but I sure as heck wouldn't ignore a possibility of catastrophic harm to a relatively delicate organ system.

Glandular therapy

The very ancient art of glandular therapy stems from almost a tribal notion that "like heals like." Although eating eyeballs won't improve your vision, this approach does have some merit when it comes to glands. Glands like the thyroid, adrenal and thymus all have appreciable levels of their constituent hormones, and in some cases, oral ingestion will in fact reasonably pass through digestion and provide the body with a significant dose of the respective hormone. This of course is provided the quality of the product is high enough and that the product is not too old in terms of shelf life.

Accepting this paradigm for a moment in the case of a sex pill, one naturally thinks of the testicles. With human testicles at a premium, one might turn to bull testicles. Originally believed to be a testosterone booster, bull testicles, also known as "orchic," have been largely available through health food stores since the late '70s.

Unfortunately, neither scientific data nor anecdotal reports seem to support use as a sex pill. I consider it at best a flimsy alternative. Although of possible use to some, dosage varies considerably from one manufacturer to another. Since there seems to be no real consensus as to how much you should take, if you really want bull testicles, I suggest you wait until you see it on a menu before you by it. That way you'll be sure, at the very least, to get a meal out of it!

Gow kee

Borrowed from the pages of TCM and also known as matrimony vine and box thorn, gow kee is a Chinese herbal medicine made from the leaves of the *lycium chinense* plant. It is well known in China as an aphrodisi-ac and male sexual aide. These apparently bland tasting leaves are finely chopped and made into a tea or eaten in raw form.

Interestingly, as legend (and I do mean legend) has it, gow kee is for male consumption only. It supposedly stimulates a man's sex drive as well as enhancing the sexual endurance of those willing consumers.

With no real studies to support it, gow kee is a bit of a stretch but still may be a solution for some.

Herb Paris

Popularized in Europe as the "love solution", herb Paris is a plant known by scientists as *Paris quadrifilia*. This narcotic shrub has long been touted as an aphrodisiac among a small circle of users. Perhaps the fact that it is a weak narcotic is the reason herb Paris has gained some notoriety as a sex pill. This seems to be evident with almost all mood-inducing substances, especially those with less prominence. It seems the mystery surrounding these "lesser knowns" adds to their seductiveness and quick mislabeling.

The main problem with herb Paris seems to be that when the bitter leaves are ingested in excess, the body reacts quite violently. The toxic response manifests itself as severe nausea and vomiting with mental status changes. Although self limited and reversible, it is not clear whether the plant is fatal in high doses.

No science or significant anecdotal reporting supports the use of herb Paris as a sex pill. In this case, and as a general caveat, I would avoid any potential death-defying feast. Otherwise, rather than finding you or your partner doubled over with pangs of ecstasy, you may well end up doubled over the toilet (not a sexy picture).

Harmel

Also known as "wild rue", *Peganum harmala* or harmel is a North African herbal medicine known to cause hallucinations. This plant is thought by ancient lore to be a sexual enhancer. Unfortunately, this mislabeling, much like the narcotics, probably stems more from its reputation as a fairly effective hallucinogenic substance. This is supported by the abuse of wild rue in southwestern United States. Native Indians and locals of Arizona, New Mexico and Texas have reportedly masticated and ingested this plant for decades purely for its mind-altering capabilities.

In short, hallucinating is no way to sexual enhancement. It is far too random an undertaking since, while at one moment you might have yourself convinced that you are at the height of sexual pleasure, the next minute you could be envisioning spiders, rats, or snakes crawling over your body. The moral of this story is that if you are going to "dice roll," I would suggest going to Vegas and not doing it with your brain.

Hormeel

Produced and distributed by a German company, hormeel is a homeopathic remedy for what seems like every sex problem known to man. This "sex panacea" is claimed by the manufacturer to help in everything from male and female fertility issues, to erectile dysfunction, to premature ejaculation, just to name a few. It is distributed in injection solution or drop form. The drops can be placed under the tongue on the order of ten drops three times each day.

Supposedly, it is a general stimulator of the endocrine system. Thus, if you have glandular problems, according to the manufacturer it is to be "...applied as a remedy for the widest variety of indications in which there is a suspicion of hormonal dysfunction." Pretty bold words, I'd say.

The fact is hormeel is a massive conglomerate of a dozen or two different ingredients. The majority of these individual substances have been minimally investigated as to effectiveness and safety. This, of course, does not mean it is not entirely possible for hormeel to work as a sexual enhancer, but it does call into question the degree of risk you take when trying it.

Apart from multivitamins, I am generally quite leery of substances with more than a few ingredients. I call it "the shot-gun effect"—just aim in the general area and blast away, crossing your fingers that you hit the target. In other words, it means putting everything, including the kitchen sink, into a formula and hoping that something in it gets the job done. I really dislike this approach because it more often than not is a signal that the product formulator is unsure of the active ingredient. When, if ever, does it make sense to combine more than a few active component ingredients? The answer, with few exceptions, is that it almost never does, unless, of course, one is attempting to hide one's ignorance.

Injection method

Although not a "sex pill" in the true sense, injectables are still an option for some and thus worth mentioning. As the billion-dollar sex pills market continues to swell (bad pun, I know), it seems that men will try virtually any method when it comes to sex. In fact, understanding the real industry growth can be viewed as directly proportional to the route of administration of sex-enhancing substances a man is willing to withstand.

In this case, the novel idea of injecting the penis to induce erection came about quite serendipitously. It seems that in 1980 a French urologic surgeon by the name of Ronald Virag accidentally anesthetized the shaft of the penis with a substance called papaverine. In much the same way Viagra or arginine work, this nitrogen-containing substance immediately resulted in a sustained erection.

The problem here is that substances like papaverine and Caverject (another prescription substance dispensed in injectable form) have proven to be tough sells to consumers simply due to the route of administration—directly injecting the penis. This has always been an obstacle for those interested. Such routes of administration can result in tissue damage and infection, not to mention the very notion of shoving a needle in your "wedding tackle" as an understandable factor limiting its use.

Jasmine

Falling into the category of aromatherapy, jasmine (an oil made from *Jasminum paniculatum*) has long been touted by proponents as a powerful aphrodisiac. As I see it, the main problem here is that, as with any aromatherapy, you never really know how much to use. After all, how much is a single dose? Is there such a thing as too much? What's good quality versus bad quality?

In addition, there is basically no clear science to aromatherapy. But don't misunderstand me. I am not saying it cannot work or that the way a substance smells doesn't effect behavior. It's just that you'll be hard pressed to find any remote science or, for that matter, even the loosest standard directives for use of this method.

In terms of using jasmine for its purported aphrodisiac qualities, it is not a pill, so don't look for exact instructions on the bottle. Instead, proponents suggest that you apply it directly on the body or inhale it from a handkerchief. There also exists the belief that by using a candle diffuser you can make the effect of inhaled jasmine last longer. In addition, some users claim it should be mixed with avocado oil for maximum effectiveness. (Sounds like a great salad dressing).

Incidentally, if all this aroma stuff is too much for you, just wait until you check out the price for pure high-quality jasmine oil extract. Bring the trust fund.

Jimsonweed

Jimsonweed, also known as *Datura stramonium* and a member of the night shade family, was traditionally used by American Indians as a stimulator of male erection. Like Spanish fly, jimsonweed is a substance that simply shouldn't be used. In fact, it is a powerful poison that can leave a person terribly sick and can easily result in fatality. Nonetheless, a vague tradition of use surrounding this compound still exists in some circles. Amid such history, sources tell me the seeds of this highly toxic plant can be ground into a fine powder and mixed with butter to form a paste. To bring out the supposed sex stimulating properties of this paste it is then eaten or smeared on the genitals.

My feeling is simple. If you try this method you will definitely be cured of any sexual dysfunction—death is quick. Even the smallest of doses can cause fatal heart rhythms and ultimately, cardiac arrest.

Kava kava

Kava kava is an herbal extract that Pacific Islanders have consumed for hundreds of years in the form of a tea drink. Proponents of the product claim it induces a state of relaxation and tranquillity. Interestingly, science seems to support its medicinal use as it has been shown in clinical studies to have muscle-relaxant, anticonvulsant and analgesic properties. In fact, many of my physician colleagues "in the know" believe it to be the most powerful anxiety eliminator available today without a prescription.

Known as a "stress soother" in Germany, it is quite popular in this country because it seems to cause less cognitive impairment (that "doe in the headlights" look) when compared with drugs like Valium or Xanax.

One might ask why a natural anxiolytic when it comes to sex? Well, for many, anxiety stands in the way of normal healthy sexual function for both men and women alike. In fact, as I see it, the irrational fear of anxiety is the single most common emotional roadblock to sexual fulfillment. If this is your only obstacle, kava may be for you.

Kwaao khruea

Fresh news from the Asian city of Bangkok, *Kwaao kruea* is an herbal remedy considered by locals to be effective for women as a beautifier and sexual aide. Specifically, it is the white variety of *Kwaao kruea* native only to specific areas of northern Thailand that has reportedly been used by local women in rural communities effectively for decades. Although these Asian women take it to strengthen hair and nails, as well as to aid in maintaining fair skin, many use it with the hopes it will make them more sexually desirable. It is said that *Kwaao kruea*, also known as pueraria mirifica, will make a woman's breasts firmer and restore a youthful female sexuality.

Interestingly, as unbelievable as these attractive claims may appear to be, this "restorative" herb is quickly gaining a fair share of attention. In fact, researchers at Bangkok's Chulalongkorn Universityas believe the herb may help stimulate estrogen production. In this way it may help women with low or waning levels of this hormone and

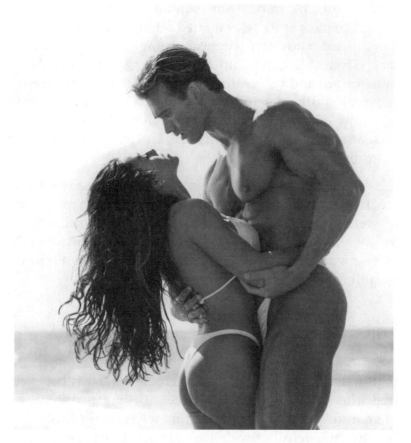

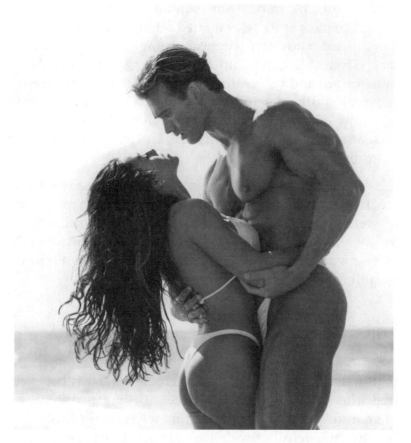

thus combat such problems as infertility, irregular menstruation and malformed breasts.

Although long-term safety issues are a concern, this fascinating herb may hold a great deal of promise in menopausal women to counter skin wrinkling, sagging breasts and bone loss. As I see it, much in the way soy and soy-based products have been touted to be "estrogen substitutes," it is quite possible that this herb may eventually prove to be effective for menopausal women that either have a problem with hormone replacement therapy or simply would rather take a chance on a natural substitute.

What Works and What Doesn't

With this in mind, one should be aware that this substance has yet to be evaluated scientifically in terms of a published study formally examining its safety and efficacy. Given this, careful attention to what we know about *Kwaao kruea* and its possible ability to act as an estrogenic agent should be carefully considered. For example, until we know more, a woman should have a healthy fear of such a substance if she has had breast cancer or if she has a strong history of the disease.

As interesting as this is, I don't see *Kwaao kruea* as being much of a "sex pill" as much as I see it as a potential rejuvenator for older women. On the other hand, who is to say that a substance that exerts such action doesn't make a woman "sexier"? Perhaps, in this way, it is a type of sex pill for women.

Lotus Seed

Lotus seed is a method occasionally recommended by both practitioners of TCM and herbologists. It is believed that the lotus seed is effective in the treatment of premature ejaculation. Unfortunately, there exists no significant scientific evidence supporting its use in this way. There is an absolute paucity of information available to date on lotus seed as it pertains to sexual enhancement, yet one still finds it mentioned periodically in the lay press.

Whether or not it has any value as a sex pill is unclear and a mechanism of action has not as of yet been elucidated (assuming one exists at all). This is in sharp contrast to yohimbine which has been shown exhaustively in the scientific literature to be effective and whose mechanism of action is both clear and well understood.

Sex Pills

I would not suggest entertaining thoughts of experimenting with lotus seed until science and reliable conventional wisdom catch up with tribal folklore.

Lycopodium

Like *Angus castus* and *Argentum nitricum, Lycopodium* is another homeopathic remedy touted by naturopathic doctors as being an aide for those with sexual dysfunction. Again, as with the other remedies mentioned, there is no scientific evidence supporting its use as a sexual enhancer for either men or women. Nor is there substantial public consensus as to its effectiveness.

Nonetheless, proponents consider it an aide for those men whose sense of apprehension limits their ability to achieve erection. It is also considered by naturopaths to be beneficial to those with premature ejaculation problems.

Interestingly, at first glance this might all sound pretty good, but on closer inspection, it simply doesn't add up. You see, in general, fear and apprehension can certainly keep you from having an erection, while over-excitation can lead to premature ejaculation. But it would be difficult and highly unlikely to have both of these problems at any one time. Consequently, it should be intuitively obvious that any substance whose proponents claim it can be used to treat both problems should immediately be viewed as suspect.

Mandrake

A member of the potato family, mandrake is the root portion of the *Mandragora officinarum*. The plant is found around the Mediterranean and has been noted since

A
B
C
D
E
F
G
H
I
J
K
L
M
N
O
P
QR
S
T
U
V
W
XYZ

ancient times for a root system that bears an uncanny resemblance to a human.

That being the case, European folklore holds that collecting the root was extremely dangerous because, when pulled from the ground, the human-like root would scream out and kill the harvester. The solution was to firmly attach meat to the plant stems and use dogs to pull out the root systems. (So much for a man's best friend).

Folklore aside, neuro-active substances have been isolated from this plant and include such potent drugs as atropine and scopolamine. These substances should intuitively cause an interference with sexual activity and impede performance. But there appears to be a psychoactive component to the substance that may contribute to a hallucinatory sensation. Beyond that, legends surrounding this substance are along the lines of magical exaggeration, but clearly potentially dangerous hocus-pocus at that.

Marijuana

"Dope", "pot", "weed", "toke", "smoke", "grass", "herb", "blunt", "ganja", or whatever you want to call it, I will refrain from over-defining marijuana to my adult readers. Obviously, given the relatively widespread use and popularity of this drug, it is almost expected that some "high seekers" have also attributed the property of sexual enhancement to its use. At first glance it almost makes intuitive sense that a substance which puts you in an altered state of relaxed consciousness might also stimulate your sexual appetite. Unfortunately, science prevails on this one in that studies on males have shown an actual decrease in sperm count, indicating a possible negative effect on testosterone (although a direct effect on lowering testosterone production has yet to be shown conclusively).

Mistletoe

It is hardly a surprise that mistletoe would find its way into a text like this one. The berries, leaves and stems of mistletoe, or *Phoradendron serotinum,* have long been thought to have some enchanting love-producing property. In addition to enhancing your sex life, folklore invests mistletoe with the ability to calm the nervous system, treat cholera and decrease bleeding after childbirth. Unfortunately, the only potentially active compounds to date isolated from this shrub are beta-phenylethylamine and tyramine. Given the innate properties of these compounds would lead one to believe mistletoe might actually be more of a stimulant for the central nervous system. In fact, from a medical standpoint, it is much more reasonable to believe that mistletoe has a greater chance of raising one's blood pressure by either a central (in the brain) mechanism or by way of its effect on the arterial system, than doing much of anything else.

Mistletoe is particularly dangerous during pregnancy and for those individuals taking monoamine-oxidase inhibitors to treat their high blood pressure. Side effects range from gastrointestinal complaints like nausea, vomiting, and diarrhea, to cardiac ramifications. Such untoward effects on the heart are of greatest concern not only in those people suffering from high blood pressure, but also possibly in those with an abnormally slow heart rhythm.

So, in terms of lovemaking, I wouldn't count on mistletoe for anything more than that "give me a kiss" trick over the doorway around Christmas time.

Mu xiang

Mu xiang, also known as "castus" or by its scientific name of *Suassurea lappa,* is a Chinese herbal substance believed to be an aphrodisiac for both men and women. The oil of the root of this plant is said to house its power. Dispensed by both Chinese herbal and Ayurvedic medicine practitioners, when taken orally this substance is broken down into specific chemicals and metabolites that are excreted in the urine. As these substances pass through the urethra (the anatomical passageway by which urine exits the body), there is an irritation of the distal orifice. The hopeful result of what is described as a painful burning sensation is an erection in men and heightened genital sensitivity in women.

Unfortunately, like so many of these less-known herbal extract preparations, there is no science to support its use. In fact, of great concern to me is the marked mechanistic similarity to Spanish fly. Thus, the same caveat comes with regard to its use. In other words—don't. The bottom-line here is that if you need pain to arouse you, forget mu xiang. I suggest leaving your genitals intact. Whips and chains might even be less dangerous.

Nitrites

The first nitrite used in wide-scale black market dealings as a sexual enhancer was amyl nitrite. Originally made as an antidote for cyanide poisoning, it was later used in inhaled form to relieve the pain of angina. Classified as an alkyl nitrite along with n-butyl nitrite, iso-butyl nitrite, iso-amyl nitrite, sec-butyl nitrite, and n-propyl nitrite, amyl nitrite is no longer made or available for any purpose in the U.S. Nonetheless, it continues to find its way into the country from foreign suppliers via the black market.

Sex Pills

The theory behind its use is that nitrites serve as almost instantaneous dilators of blood vessels. In so doing, without too much mind-bending one can understand how, by way of this mechanism of action, they might be used not only for getting more blood to the heart, but for increasing supply to the genitals as well. Add to that, nitrites and nitrite derivatives seem to be quite effective in dilating sphincters anywhere in the body. (I'll let your imagination work on that one).

One of the biggest problems with early use of substances like amyl nitrite and the reason far better substances have taken its place has to do with route of entry. These nitrites were sealed in delicate glass capsules housed by foamy nets. With a slight bend, the capsule was broken, releasing the liquid contents into the surrounding absorptive casing. The entire casing was then placed under the nose for immediate inhaling. It should be plain to see how dosage would be difficult to control. After all, it would simply depend on technique: how well you break the inner capsule; how deeply you inhale; how close in proximity to your nose you put the casing; and the confluence of your nasal passageway all factor in to the amount of chemical you deliver into your body. With such an inconsistent method of delivery, it's not surprising that such a drug would quickly become obsolete in our current climate of rapidly advancing medicine.

In short, the "skinny" on such nitrites is pure and simple. They are extremely dangerous if taken by an individual overly sensitive to its action. With unpredictable dose delivery rapidly dilating the arteries and suddenly increasing blood flow, a reactive speeding up of the heart (also known as reflex tachycardia) results. This reaction can be quite detrimental and even fatal to a sensitive heart.

Simply stated, for a sex pill I suggest looking elsewhere since, although you might be in for a thrill, it might not end up being the one you had in mind.

Nutmeg

This interesting spice has long been endowed with aphrodisiac qualities. Also known by its scientific name *Myristica fragrans,* nutmeg is produced from the Myristicaceae tree. The seeds of the tree are stripped of coat, dried, and ground into a fine powder.

Unlike so many other spices endowed with unreal and imagined qualities, nutmeg as a sex pill may have some credence, albeit attributable to an indirect quality. It seems that nutmeg, although not directly an aphrodisiac, does have hallucinogenic properties. Specifically, the chemical myristicin has a hallucinogenic effect similar to that of mescaline (derived from the peyote cactus) and is found in unusually high concentration in nutmeg. Thus, it has actually developed a reputation in prisons as a way to "get high" when the limits of incarceration make black market underground drugs hard to come by.

Whether or not such a "buzz" can constitute a sex pill, there remains a distinct warning to the abuser. In even the slightest excess, nutmeg is considered potentially dangerous by many experts as it can exert a seemingly unpredictable effect on the central nervous system and on cardiovascular stability.

I suggest using nutmeg to season foods, but not to stimulate one's sexual appetite.

Orchid root

When orchid roots are gathered, dried and boiled, the result is a substance referred to as "salep". Usually a collection of several different species of orchid root, salep originated in the 18th century as an aphrodisiac and sexual enhancer. The reason was believed to center around the notion that the root structure resembled human testicles in much the same way fenugreek was believed to resemble the human phallus and thus yield aphrodisiac properties. In fact, the Arab transliteration is "saleb," meaning fox testicles.

Traditionally, orchid root is prepared by boiling the root collection with substances like milk, cinnamon, cloves, ginger, and/or parsnip if you're Swedish.

In short, I'd pass on the gruel.

Pepper

Used by the ancient Egyptians, Arabs, Greeks, Romans, and Indians, pepper can be found in many forms. From fresh to dried or preserved, from ripe to unripe, it is a versatile spice with a plethora of well-founded and not so well-founded uses. Beyond its reputation as a widely popular spice and flavoring, pepper, or *Piper nigrum,* has also been called an aphrodisiac for both men and women. Legend has it that doing everything from sprinkling it on your body, to rubbing it on the male genitalia, to even drinking it with milk and nuts will result in the desired effect of heightened sexual pleasure.

Although chavicine, a relatively unique active compound, has been isolated from pepper, scientists believe that this substance is responsible for little more than the strong aroma and taste. Having nothing to do with sexual enhancement, chavicine along with several other natural chemicals contribute to the pungency of the spice.

How pepper ever got labeled a possible aphrodisiac is a mystery. To add to the confusion, it seems old-world Europeans used to refer to spices in general and mixtures of several spices as peppers. This raises a question as to whether actual pepper, or perhaps some other substance, was really the aphrodisiac.

Either way, forget pepper as a sex pill. It's not likely to stimulate anything more than your taste buds.

Potency wood

Also known as *Muira puama,* potency wood is a plant native to Brazil. It has been used for hundreds of years by South Americans as a folk medicine and aphrodisiac. In particular, improvement in libido and male sexual function are among the claims of users. Unfortunately, so little is known about this substance that it has failed to get much press. In fact, it is almost always overlooked as a therapeutic agent.

Interestingly, research does seem to lend a little support to its use as a sex pill. A 1990 study conducted at the Institute of Sexology in France looked at 262 males with decreased libido as well as those with erectile dysfunction. sixty-two percent of those suffering from a low libido showed improvement, while fifty-one percent of those men with erectile dysfunction felt they improved. Although not a particularly well-designed study, it does seem to point to some benefit of potency wood.

Given the relative paucity of information available on this substance and the fact that it is not readily available to the consumer, I don't generally recommend it. Nonetheless, it is something you should know about. With time, it may prove to be a viable and effective sex pill.

Pygeum africanum

In the area of urology, *Pygeum africanum,* a botanical extract produced from powdered tree bark, has been fairly well studied, and in fact, has been proven to improve a man's ability to achieve and sustain an erection. Although several studies have been done, one in particular stands out. Patients with benign prostatic hypertrophy or prostatitis, suffering erectile dyfunction, were given pygeum africanum in a double blind fashion. Erectile activity was measured during sleep using penile tumescence. Amazingly, despite the ability of these diseases to interfere with erectile function, the group taking the *Pygeum africanum* showed a clear improvement over placebo.

Understand that normal prostate secretion is essential for fertility. In addition, proper function of muscular bands coursing through the prostate probably governs the fertility function and subsequent sensation of the male ejaculation. *Pygeum africanum* has been shown in clinical trials to increase prostatic secretion and improve the composition of seminal fluid. In particular, pygeum africanum led to increased levels of seminal fluid and a healthier make-up of its components (i.e., alkaline phosphatase).

Ricin

Ricin is made from the seeds of the castor oil plant, otherwise known as *Ricinus communis.* In the days when hell hath no fury like my grandmother's wrath, castor oil was used as a punishment and purgative. So, how did anyone end up using it as an aphrodesiac? Well, according to Johan's Guide to Aphrodesiacs, it would seem to be due to a "linguistic mistake".

Supposedly, the Latin etymology of ricinus refers to a tick. This was a descriptive effort in ancient times to describe the seeds of the *Ricinus communis* as resembling the shape of a swollen tick. This apparently led to the Swedish interpretation of the label as being "tyckfro." The problem here is that, although descriptively similar, the literal meaning of the word in Swedish is "affection seed".

Thus, the delusion-filled madness of ingesting this purgative as an aphrodisiac began. Does it work? Well, if sticking your finger down your throat and vomiting makes you horny, it could quite possibly work for you. But if your physiology resembles most other humans on this planet, I suggest passing. Somehow, I just don't see the titillation in blowing the dust off grandma's old punishment cocktail and calling it a sex pill.

Royal jelly

Royal jelly is a thick milky substance that is secreted from the pharyngeal glands of bees in their sixth and twelfth days of life. It is naturally created when honey and pollen are combined. Royal jelly contains many vitamins and minerals, including all of the B-complex vitamins as well as enzymes, hormones, amino acids, antibacterial agents and antibiotic substances.

Royal jelly is believed by many to make the immune system stronger. While it is viewed by some as a sexual enhancer and is found in several sex pills, its reputation has been built on Asian folklore. There isn't a scrap of data to support its use for such purposes.

Sex Pills

Actual royal jelly spoils easily. In order to preserve it, it must be kept tightly sealed and in a refrigerator. Worse yet, in a select unlucky few, royal jelly has been linked to asthma attacks, allergic reactions and even death. So, especially if you're allergic to bees, look out!

Saffron

Saffron lists in the category of a spice. This pricy orange condiment is derived from parts of the *Crocus sativus* plant. It is commonly described as a bitter spice with a sharp flavor that you either love or hate. Saffron has been used sparingly for ages in both Asian and European cooking as primarily a seafood and soup spice. Pure fresh saffron is expensive and rare.

By a means not entirely clear, saffron somehow gained a limited reputation as an aphrodisiac. Ingesting saffron is said to make the genitals more sensitive to stimulation. True or not, no actual active compound that can be directly linked to a sex-stimulating effect has been isolated in the spice. The substances "crocin" (considered to give saffron its unusual color) and "picrocrocin" (considered responsible for its taste) have both been isolated, but neither chemical is believed to have any activity as an aphrodisiac. In addition, there exist no reliable reports supporting any effect whatsoever on genital sensitivity in either men or women.

It is quite possible that the weaker qualities of the human psyche as much as anything else are to blame for saffron's false reputation as an aphrodisiac. It is the uniquely human tendency to take substances that are rare in our earthly domain and, simply because of their scarcity, attach magical and almost divine qualities to these otherwise humble and often near-extinct substances.

It is perplexing to consider why simply a paucity of a substance is oftentimes enough to make everyone want to possess it, despite a lack of any true intrinsically redeeming qualities. Nonetheless, it remains one of man's most peculiar habits to identify something as rare or expensive and then eat it, kill it, wear it, or hang it in a trophy case.

Sarsaparilla

Traditionally Mexican and South-American in origin, sarsaparilla is a general name for the different preparations from the *Smilax* species, depending the area of the globe. The roots of this plant are gathered, dried, powdered or chopped, and boiled to make an aphrodisiac potion.

In this case, as "loopy" as it might sound, this particular plant preparation may be quite real and effective. Historically, sarsaparilla was used in the 18th century as a treatment for syphilis. The fact is, there is real medicinal value to this root. Perhaps of even greater interest is that its active ingredients have been isolated and include sarasponin and saraspogenin. It is these isolated substances that closely resemble sex hormones in structure. Perhaps these hormones directly stimulate receptors in our bodies or convert to hormones that our bodies recognize to regulate libido.

Although this points to a very real potential efficacy, these "sterol" substances more closely resemble proges-terone and pregnenolone than testosterone. Thus, the formation of an excess of the female sex hormone estrogen is a very real and unwanted possibility.

Until more research is done, perhaps the best role for sarsaparilla remains as a flavoring agent in root beer.

Sex Pills

Saw palmetto

Saw palmetto *(Serona repens)* is a substance extracted from the berries of a palm tree commonly found throughout Florida. Often mislabeled and misused as a libido enhancer, it is a substance that is used very effectively to alleviate benign prostatic hypertrophy in older males. Saw palmetto has been clinically tested and shown to effectively decrease the symptoms associated with prostate enlargement. In fact, a recent study conducted at the University of Chicago involving 50 men with benign prostatic hypertrophy, found that the group taking the saw palmetto experienced nearly 50% improvement in their urinary symptoms.

While not a common cause of erectile dysfunction, the bladder-relieving problems and urinary symptoms associated with benign prostatic hypertrophy can interfere with intercourse. In addition, an enlarged prostate can interfere with nerves and blood vessels feeding the penis. In an effort to avoid risky surgery, drugs like Proscar are frequently prescribed to help alleviate the urinary symptoms. The problem with these drugs is that they often actually cause erectile dysfunction or a loss of sexual desire in the men who take them.

Interestingly, an effective way of avoiding benign prostatic hypertrophy is to engage in regular and fairly frequent sexual activity. It seems that by attaining erection and, ultimately, contraction of the muscular bands throughout the prostate during ejaculation, you in effect bring greater blood flow to this region. Greater blood flow and circulation means increased oxygen and nutrient delivery to this area, which is essential to proper organ function and health.

In short, saw palmetto is best used as a prostate health supplement for men over the age of forty and is not, by itself, a libido enhancer. But if your problem centers around benign prostatic hypertrophy, it may have great potential as a sex pill.

Shellfish

Although hardly fitting the definition of sex pills by any stretch of meaning, shellfish are still worth mentioning in the context of the subject simply because of the considerable legend and lore attached to these creatures. Lobsters, oysters, clams, and a host of other shellfish have been incorrectly labeled as aphrodisiacs.

Oysters in particular have long been considered powerful sexual enhancers. In fact, dating back to the 17th century an offering of oysters was considered a clear signal of sexual "interest". Some claim that it is the zinc content that is responsible for the effect. Since I don't believe oysters are an aphrodisiac any more than I believe zinc contributes anything, I think shellfish are nothing more than a great appetizer. Sorry to spoil the romance.

Shiitake

Also known as *Lentinula edodes,* the shiitake is a large mushroom popular throughout Asia and rapidly gaining recognition as a medicinal plant in America. It can be cooked or eaten dry and has a curiously delicious smoky flavor. Studied at the University of Michigan, shiitake was found to have an active ingredient called "lentinan" which can apparently significantly stimulate the immune system. It is said to work as an effective antiviral by increasing interferon activity. In keeping with this, a

Japanese study found that shiitake was actually better than the drug amantadine for the treatment of viral illness. In addition, some studies allude to shiitake being a possible cholesterol-lowering agent.

Science has provided no support for shiitake as an aphrodisiac. However, for those who still believe in the sex-enhancing powers of shiitake, it is rumored that shiitake should be eaten in combination with game for greatest effectiveness.

Apart from what appear to be unfounded wives tales and loose testimony at best, in terms of shiitake being an aphrodisiac, it should be noted that this substance does deserve a great deal of attention for other purposes. The scientific community seems to agree with me on this, as there are a number of studies currently underway in both Japan and the U.S. looking at possible medicinal and scientific uses of shiitake.

Spanish Fly

Spanish fly (also known as cantheride) is an extract from the Mediterranean meloid beetle. This "love potion" has been made for hundreds of years by crushing these beetles into a fine powder and ingesting it prior to intercourse.

Popularized in the bygone "Studio 54" era of sexual promiscuity, Spanish fly is used by both men and women. It works by producing what is described as a burning sensation in the penis and vagina. Unfortunately, and despite the rumors, beyond this warm genital sensation, it does nothing to enhance erection. In fact, women often experience a painful mucosal irritation that can lead to ulcerative abrasions and subsequent serious infection. Worse yet, it is considered a poison and can cause irreparable damage to both the kidneys and gastrointestinal tract.

Add to that, the *American Journal of Emergency Medicine* reported a number of cases of users with complaints that ranged from severe abdominal pain, mouth burning and vomiting to bleeding and pain upon urination.

It is illegal in the United States, but sex shops reportedly still routinely distribute the substance in black market fashion. Simply stated, it is a dangerous substance that should be avoided at all cost.

St. John's wort

St. John's wort (also known as *Hypericum perforatum*) is an herbal remedy that dates back hundreds of years. Traditionally, it is harvested in the summer and used as a heal-all, for inflammatory conditions in particular. In more recent years it has emerged as a treatment for anxiety and depression.

Classically referred to as "the herb that lifts the spirit," recent scientific studies seem to support the efficacy of St. John's wort. In fact, a meta-analysis of 23 separate trials all comparing St. John's wort with placebo and/or antidepressant drugs, showed fairly conclusively that the herb was beneficial in cases of mild to moderate depression.

Although its effect on positively modulating mood cannot be refuted, the fact is it has never been shown to enhance sexual desire or performance. Nonetheless, people still buy it, hoping it will help.

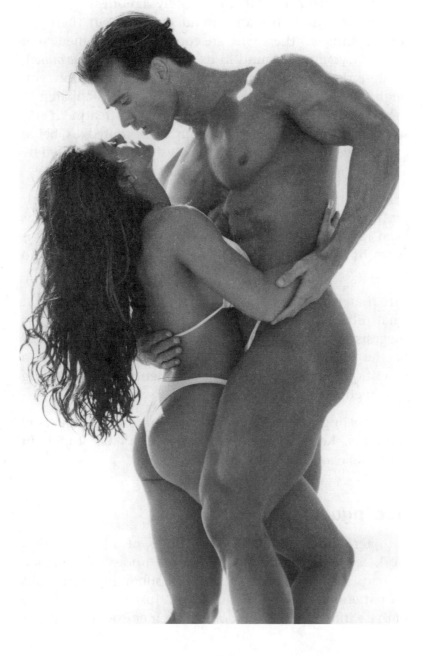

What Works and What Doesn't

Strychnine

Hard to believe that this deadly colorless, odorless crystalline poison has any useful purpose, but there are homeopaths out there who are convinced it has medicinal value. Strychnos is found in its natural form *"nux vomica"* (quite a descriptive euphemism if you consider how you might feel after ingestion—like vomiting). It is apparently used by these "bold" practitioners as a treatment for sexual dysfunction. In particular, it is touted as being extremely effective if one's sexual dysfunction is caused by alcohol, cigarette smoking, or dietary problems.

If all this sounds peculiar to you, I share your sentiments. Somehow I can't see taking a body that has been ravaged with alcohol or cigarettes and poisoning it again in hopes of making it "better." It simply makes no sense.

If that isn't disturbing enough for you, consider that what little literature on the use of strychnine exists suggests "only seeing a practitioner experienced in the use" of the substance. My only question is, how does a practitioner gain this so-called experience without killing some people along the way?

My feelings are to stay far away from esoteric snake-oil solutions. Keep an open mind but don't be stupid. In short, take a pass on the strychnine.

Sublingual method

In terms of fast action, few routes of administration work as well as sublingual (dissolved under the tongue). Perhaps the best example is that of sublingual nitro tabs for patients with anginal chest pain. Just observe any one of these individuals during one of their episodes and you'll witness first hand the power and efficiency of this method of drug delivery. So it makes sense that this method is being so heavily investigated by the sex pill industry. It is a powerful, quick, easy and relatively noninvasive means of administering a substance.

A rather large Japanese company is working on a fast acting sublingual form of the injectable drug Vasomax. Also known as "phentolamine," and like its injectable counterpart, sublingual delivery also works on the principle of dilating blood vessels and increasing blood flow to the penis. Problems here are that the drug is not yet available and, once distributed, will require a prescription from your doctor.

Testosterone can also be delivered sublingually. Some companies showcase this method because it bypasses the digestive action of the gastrointestinal tract. The thing to keep in mind is that again, it is a pharmaceutical substance that you need a prescription for.

If a more natural, non-prescription method is more to your liking, there is a product called Vitalin T. It is a sublingual spray form of androstenedione. Although it is marketed as a long-term testosterone booster, as you know from reading my section on androstenedione, I think its best chance is to work as a short-term libido enhancer.

Suppository Method

When one hears the word "suppository," an interesting response is usually evoked, namely, an emotionally charged "not me!" Perhaps this is a product of the conditioned response to the traditional suppository route of administration—the rectum. But, in this case, I speak not of tail with no tail, but rather of the head with no brain!

This interesting method of inducing erection is the penile suppository route. As disconcerting as that might sound, it is a rather efficient route of administration whereby the drug enters locally at its site of action. The problem with this method is that many men complain of a burning sensation after its use that at times can be quite severe.

There is a product available with a prescription called "Muse" that works much like Caverject by dilating penile blood vessels. It also is quite effective, but you just have to get comfy with the concept of "pecker pellets"—not a cozy thought, if you ask me.

Testosterone

Testosterone is the male sex hormone. It is a powerful steroid molecule with both anabolic and androgenic characteristics. As an anabolic, it has the ability to govern and promote tissue recovery and muscle building, and thus has been primarily used in the bodybuilding and sports world as a recovery, performance-enhancing, and muscle-building aide. As an androgenic, it controls the secondary male sex characteristics including hair growth, deepening of the voice, aggression, and perhaps of greatest importance in the context of this book, sex drive.

In recent years there have been strong efforts in research to modify the structure of the testosterone molecule in order to come up with testosterone derivatives that minimize androgenicity while preserving or maximizing the anabolic component. The reason is that for therapeutic purposes in patients with specific problems (i.e., anemia or renal insufficiency, severe burns, wasting diseases like AIDS or some types of cancer, etc.), it is the anabolic tissue rebuilding and recuperative aspects that are of clinical value, not the androgenic component that is of interest. The androgenic index is the aspect considered to have unwanted side effects and thus, to be avoided.

Since testosterone derivatives are more anabolic and less androgenic, making them appropriate for the populations mentioned, they are nearly ineffective when it comes to enhancing sex drive. This is again due to the fact that it is the androgenic component that governs libido. Without a significant androgenic component, as is the case with the testosterone derivatives, you have no hope of stimulating libido. For that, the more appropriate solution is pure testosterone.

In men with a low libido and a low level of bioavailable testosterone or free testosterone, hormone replacement therapy to enhance sexual desire works well. A steroid with such androgenic activity is appropriate in cases of what is called "primary hypogonadism" or in those suffering "hypogonadotropic hypogonadism." There may be other select cases of individuals in need of libido enhancement with testosterone therapy, but this is a very small sub-population of patients and it should only be given at the discretion of a physician. In fact, it is a widely held belief that, with the exception of true hypogonadal males, testosterone therapy offers little more than placebo benefit.

On the other hand, given my own clinical experience coupled with the poorly-defined wide reference range of normal testosterone levels for the healthy adult male, I am of the strong belief that the introduction of a higher level of free testosterone in a subject with a "normal" level can in many individuals result in a strong stimulation of libido.

What Works and What Doesn't

Unfortunately, apart from the injectable and transdermal testosterones, the oral analog (known as Halotestin) has numerous possible side effects which include, among other things, serious liver problems. This limits widespread use and should be a strong motivator to try something more natural. If a sex pill is all you're interested in, when it comes to testosterone, you may be biting off more than you had hoped.

Topical cream method

Although not oral pills, topical formulas including prostaglandin and papaverine creams are currently being researched and thus worth mentioning. Applied to the surface of the genitals, these creams also operate on the principle of locally stimulating blood flow. In women, testosterone cream has been used for augmentation of sexual responsiveness. Some clinicians recommend vaginal testosterone cream for young women with decreased libido.

My feeling about topical formulations is quite basic. Be aware that they are useful options for both men and women, but I don't see them as ever becoming very popular when one can simply ingest a prescription or natural non-prescription pill and get the same or better effect.

Tribulus terrestrus

Tribulus terrestrus is an herbal supplement growing in popularity within the bodybuilding circle as a testosterone stimulator. Whether true or not, proponents site a rather obscure Bulgarian use patent as evidence of its efficacy. In theory, tribulus terrestrus is supposedly what we call an "LH analog". LH is the abbreviation for leutinizing hormone. LH is produced by cells in the anterior of the pituitary gland (an endocrine gland located in the center of the brain near the base of the skull). In males, LH stimulates the interstitial cells of Leydig located in the testicles to produce testosterone.

The true proven analog of LH is human chorionic gonadotropin or "HCG". HCG is produced by the placenta and is extracted from a pregnant woman's urine. It is a powerful prescription medication that acts like LH and stimulates the production of testosterone.

Tribulus terrestrus, on the other hand, is thought of by the bodybuilding community as sort of a poor man's HCG. It is taken with the hope of boosting the body's own production of testosterone. Whether this makes for a sex pill is questionable. For one thing, we are not yet sure from a scientific standpoint if tribulus terrestrus can really boost testosterone. Of course, if this is the case, then certainly a libido enhancement would be a logical effect. Also, if it can boost testosterone, I could see it as possibly effective as a general sexual health formula for the so-called "andropausal" males (assuming you believe that males have their own version of menopause). But keep in mind, despite the hype you read, it simply hasn't been proven yet. As a sex pill this substance doesn't get a lot of recognition from me because even if it does work to stimulate testosterone production, it will only help you over the long haul, primarily exerting its effect only after being taken chronically. This is because the theoretical mechanism of action is so slow.

Lastly, we must consider safety issues, especially given a substance we know so little about and whose proponents recommend a chronic dosing pattern. Assuming I have been a good and responsible steward of this text, you should know that "natural" and "herbal" in origin are not synonyms for health. In fact, as you should recognize from the many substances covered in this text, a natural herbal supplement can also make you sick or even kill you. So, bottom line, although interesting, the jury is still out on tribulus terrestrus.

Truffles

This vegetable aphrodisiac was originally popularized in ancient Rome as a way to conjure up sexual feelings. Ancient writings of the time make reference to a myriad of ways to prepare truffle delicacies. Truffles remained popular in Rome as different types were rated in terms of strength and efficacy. Of course, Rome burned and along with it, the truffle craze went up in smoke.

Enter the late 1700s, when truffle "magic" was revisited by the French. With the Parisians adding their own unique flair, the reputation of the truffle took on mythical proportions. With the power of romantic legend heaped upon this puny botanical, truffle use swept throughout Europe and Great Britain.

Heaven knows how the legend of the truffle has survived the ages, but perhaps, like tarot cards or palm reading, the idea that truffles contain some power as an aphrodisiac is simply timeless. Maybe it's the "forbidden fruit" idea. Unfortunately, that doesn't necessarily make it true. There is absolutely no science to back its use. Simply stated, I wouldn't count on truffles to spark sex, but I'd be willing to bet they make great soup.

Unicorn root

Unicorn root, also known as *Aletrius farinosa,* is an herbal medicinal remedy used in cases of impotence. In

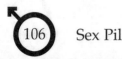

addition, it has also been classically recommended for cases of benign prostatic hypertrophy. Interestingly, it apparently is so effective for cases of impotence that it has been used as a fertility agent and sexual enhancer for both men and women. It is in the relative uniqueness of unisex activity whereby this substance poses an advantage over many other sex pills.

Although anecdotally the support for this substance as a sex pill is fairly significant, there is a complete lack of scientific research to support its use. The main problem here for me is simply one of safety. I generally like to see at least a single significant research study supporting the safe use of a substance over time to minimally ease my concerns. The facts are simply that there are no facts to support its safe use.

Vacuum method

Another non-pill method worthy of mentioning is vacuum erection therapy. This technology was invented in 1961 by Geddings Osbon, himself a sufferer of erectile dysfunction. In an effort to recapture his ability to achieve erection, Osbon "tooled around" and came up with his solution. The result was a rather "Austin Powers-esque" method of blowing the dust off his family jewels. He had invented the world's first vacuum device for erectile dysfunction.

This unique, non-invasive and drug free method of inducing erection works by placing a plastic cylinder over the shaft of the penis and then creating a negative pressure via a pump. The action will cause blood to rush into the penis in response to the external pressure. Interestingly, this method works regardless of the source of a man's erection problem.

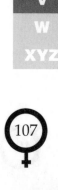

In general, this method is considered quite safe and is frequently recommended by urologists to patients following prostate surgery. Nonetheless, no method is without its downside. In this case, overuse can result in erectile tissue damage and penile discoloration and numbness.

Valerian

Valerian, or *Valeriana officinalis,* is yet another product that, like kava kava, is enormously popular in Europe for the treatment of anxiety. In fact, it is also approved in Europe for the treatment of insomnia and other sleep disorders. Statistics show over 50 tons of valerian are consumed in France every year. Unfortunately, unlike kava, there are really no impressive significant scientific studies of valerian in either the United States or Europe. However, the anecdotal reports are literally overwhelming in support of its use.

One small-scale study on Hispanic women under treatment for a variety of psychiatric disorders including major depression, anxiety, and insomnia in an urban community found that the women's conditions subjectively improved.

These observations lend credence to the utility of valerian as a hypnotic and mood enhancer. Again, like kava, if anxiety is an issue for you as it pertains to standing in the way of healthy sexual relations, valerian could prove effective.

Vanilla

Here, I don't speak of the vanilla of ice cream fame, but rather the pure North American wild vanilla as it occurs in nature, also known as *Trisila odoratissima*. Of course, just because the latter sounds a bit more exotic, that shouldn't compel you to think it is any more effective for enhancing sex than a Ben and Jerry's dessert concoction.

At any rate, the conventional wisdom seems to be that in the early to mid- 1900s, wild vanilla was used to treat malaria. Although unsuccessful in having any effect on containing the disease, exotic, erotic, and sexually vivid dreams were an apparent side effect of the treatment.

True or not, there is no scientific support here and the small number of people that reported this side effect came from a clearly limited sub-population of individuals in numbers too few to make any general inferences. Even if true, I think most of us would prefer a sexually explicit life experience to a sexually explicit dream.

On the other hand, there is traditional vanilla. It is commonly found in the spice or deodorizing section of the grocery store shelf. Cured from the orchid plant vanilla plantifolia, this deliciously pungent plant extract was considered to be a sex stimulant throughout much of Europe in the 1800's. Currently, proponents claim vanilla has a natural love-arousing effect in both men and women. They say the positive effects are derived as much from the odor as from the taste, but I caution against using inferior synthetic products as they apparently lack the potency of the natural substance.

Whether nontraditional or traditional, synthetic or natural, I can't realistically see vanilla as a sex pill of any kind. Nonetheless, my mother makes great use of it when cooking and I like the vanilla air fresheners for my closet. Other than that, I'd have to say that that the rumors about vanilla being some kind of aphrodisiac are just that—rumors.

Vasomax

Vasomax, also called "phentolamine", is an experimental oral version of an already approved injectable drug. Developed by Schering-Plough and Zonagen, it is a reformulation of an old blood pressure medication. Like the injectable, the oral form works by blocking the neurotransmitter norepinephrine. The result is a dilating of blood vessels and increased blood flow to the penis. The experimental oral form works via the same proposed mechanism. Male trials are near completion here in the U.S., while female trials are in the planning stages.

The bottom line on this sex pill is that the jury is still out in terms of its effectiveness and safety. In particular, one should be concerned about a possible rapid and precipitous fall in blood pressure if Vasomax is taken in excess or simply ingested by an individual exquisitely sensitive to the substance.

Viagra

It's been all over the papers. It's been on nearly every news program. Called "Viagra," it's the latest pharmaceutical fascination. From the moment this drug met with FDA approval, the lines have been forming at doctors' offices around the country with men eager to try this latest rage. Needless to say, there is quite a bit of excitement (no pun intended) surrounding this new drug.

Sex Pills

Viagra, known to scientists as "sildenafil citrate" or "Viagra UK-92480," was officially approved on March 27, 1998, by the FDA as an erectile response enhancer. This drug, only available with a doctor's prescription, was originally developed as a heart medication. It was found to incidentally stimulate erection in those taking it. The drug has been studied for the past five years as a treatment for men who have difficulty achieving erections due to, or as a consequence of, conditions like diabetes, vascular disease or spinal cord injury, and cancer patients who have undergone radical prostatectomy. It should be noted, however, that those men with no apparent organic cause for their impotence seem to do the best.

To comprehend how it works, one must begin with an understanding of a little anatomy and physiology. Simply stated, in order to achieve erection, one must begin with proper "parasympathetic" nerve stimulation (see figure 9).

Neurologic response patterns are governed by two general "systems". The first is the sympathetic nervous system. It is often referred to as a "fight or flight" mechanism and is activated in times of intense emotions like aggression, fear, pain, or extreme exhilaration. The physiologic results are seen in the form of a fast heart rate, increased blood pressure, dilated pupils, and decreased stomach activity. On the contrary, the parasympathetic nervous system is referred to as the "rest and digest" mechanism. When activated by feelings or situations like calm, quiet, and safety, the physiologic results are things like slower pulse rate, decreased blood pressure, pin-point pupils, and increased stomach activity.

A male needs both systems intact to engage in intercourse and achieve orgasm. Relative to the neurologic mechanisms, the parasympathic (or "rest and digest")

system controls arousal, initial erection, and the maintenance of erection. In other words, if you can't get into a relaxed state of mind, forget trying to have or keep an erection because it won't happen. The parasympathetic system maintains control of normal sexual function throughout the sexual act and up until the point of ejaculation, at which time the sympathetic system takes over to achieve orgasm.

Thus, it is essential to have proper parasympathetic stimulation for male arousal. In other words, you had better be "in the mood" and relaxed enough to achieve erection, or forget it.

So, assuming the proper relaxing parasympathetic nerve stimulation is present, blood will rush into "pockets" within the shaft of the penis known as the "corpus cavernosum". The result of blood entering the shaft is an enlargement and stiffening of the penis. Regulation of blood filling the corpus cavernosum is governed by nitric oxide production. An increase in nitric oxide concentration in the corpus cavernosum activates an enzyme called guanylate cyclase. Activation of this enzyme results in an increase in the production of a chemical called cGMP. It is the cGMP that directly relaxes blood vessels and allows them to expand. The result is that blood rushes into the shaft of the penis.

Almost immediately following the production of cGMP, another compound called cGMP phosphodiesterase is activated. This chemical, also known as PDE-5, breaks down cGMP as fast as it is formed. The result of the destruction of cGMP by PDE-5 is a decrease in smooth muscle relaxation and blood flow to the penis. Subsequently, erection is terminated.

"Mechanism of Action of PDE-5 in Terminating Erection:"

Phosphodiesterase 5 (PDE-5)

↓

Cyclic Guanosine Monophosphate (cGMP) Production ▌ ⟶ Smooth Muscle Relaxation

in the Corpus Cavernosum ⟶ Increased Blood Flow to the Penis

The PDE-5 enzyme is selectively and temporarily blocked by Viagra. At the molecular level, Viagra is a highly selective and very potent inhibitor of PDE-5, such that when present, it will effectively inhibit this enzyme system. This allows cGMP to remain in high concentration and build-up in the corpus cavernosum. The end result is that blood will more easily fill the corpus cavernosum and, with the proper stimulation, erection should be more easily achieved and maintained.

"Mechanism of Inhibition of PDE-5 by Viagra:"

Phosphodiesterase 5 (PDE-5)

↓

▬ Viagra

↓

Cyclic Guanosine Monophosphate (cGMP) Production ⟶ Smooth Muscle Relaxation

in the Corpus Cavernosum ⟶ Increased Blood Flow to the Penis

Viagra has been demonstrated to have a rapid absorption and a relatively short half-life (the shorter the half-life, the less time a substance stays in the body). Maximum blood concentrations are reached in about 60 minutes.

Keep in mind that Viagra does not directly cause penile erections and has no effect in the absence of sexual stimulation. In fact, in a clinical study of 12 patients with erectile dysfunction Viagra was shown to specifically enhance the erectile response to visual sexual stimulation. This implies that Viagra aids only in the excitatory phase but has no effect on enhancing your desire for sex or on staving off ejaculation once past the arousal phase.

Also, remember that Viagra is a prescription medication and is not without side effects. In particular, the most common complaints are headache, facial flushing and indigestion. The FDA also notes that 3% of men taking Viagra reported changes in their vision (in particular, an alteration in the perception of color). In addition, although there appears to be virtually no effect on the heart or blood pressure, the FDA warns against taking the drug with any nitrate-based cardiac medications (i.e., sublingual nitroglycerin tablets, nitroglycerin patches, etc.), as the drug acts by enhancing the smooth muscle relaxing effects of nitric oxide (a chemical released in response to sexual stimulation). A combination might result in a significant and potentially dangerous drop in blood pressure.

Of greatest concern are the nearly 200 deaths reported in the first year attributed either directly or indirectly to the use of Viagra. In fact, in the first four months alone after the product came to market, there were 69 reported fatalities. Of course, most of these men were over the age of 60 and at least 46 had heart problems. Some were taking nitrates. Subsequently, the producer has warned that the combination of Viagra with nitrates can result in death. But the same manufacturer insists that Viagra did not by itself cause a single death. They think it's safe, but of course they sell it.

Perhaps the biggest concern, as it pertains to the studies done on Viagra, is the relatively limited number of study

Sex Pills

participants. This critique centers on the fact that the absolute numbers of men that took part in the studies is quite low when compared with the unanticipated widespread use of the drug. The problem here is that some adverse reactions may be revealed only when large numbers of people are observed taking the substance.

If you're just a "recreational" user and you don't suffer from erectile dysfunction, distributor consumer information tells us not to make the mistake of thinking that Viagra is going to further "juice up" an already normal sex life. As explained, based on the mechanism at work, the fundamental activity in bona fide cases of erectile dysfunction appears to be an overzealous or early breakdown of cGMP. Distributors believe men with no such imbalance will likely have normal nitric oxide and cGMP levels. Given this, the thinking is that if you don't truly suffer from erectile dysfunction, you are not going to see any difference in erections (except perhaps when you check your wallet and see how much you spent for a single pill—observe how quickly "turned off" you become). Unfortunately, conventional wisdom tells us the contrary. Sometimes, men who don't have erectile dysfunction get hold of Viagra and claim it does, in fact, further enhance their sexual abilities. The same "word on the street" holds for women despite the fact that it is not yet approved for female consumption.

At any rate, if you are interested, the recommended dose is 50 mg taken an hour before sex. Keep in mind that some people require more (up to 100 mg) or less (only 25 mg) to generate the desired response. This drug should also not be used more than once a day and, in my opinion, only under the direction of your physician. It will cost any-where from $7 to about $10 per pill, and this cost is likely to continue to climb. In fact, my friends in Europe and

Asia tell me that the black market demand for the little blue pills can exceed a price of $40 apiece.

An interesting aside to this drug is its potential efficacy in women. As the medical field begins to learn more about male impotence and its management, my physician colleagues are increasingly convinced the underlying mechanism of sexual dysfunction in males and females may not be so far apart. That being the case, Viagra trials in the female population are already under way in Europe. Currently the FDA is considering approving testing of the drug in females here in the U.S. The theory is based on the fact that the clitoris is the female "version" of the penis, both from an embryonic standpoint and, to some degree, from a functional perspective (it similarly becomes engorged with blood during sexual arousal). However, as a practical physician, my only question is how the heck are these researchers going to measure this female arousal? I wonder if my male brethren scientists have considered this perplexity. It should be interesting to see how they figure it out.

Wellbutrin

Wellbutrin was originally developed in the U.S. as an antidepressant. Although not a very popular antide-pressant medication among practitioners, Wellbutrin had the distinction of being one of the only drugs of this type not to depress sex drive. In fact, the company found that it actually stimulated libido in those taking it. In addition, according to the manufacturer, unlike other types of antidepressent medications, Wellbutrin is also free of sedative and blood pressure side effects.

Unfortunately, the effects of Wellbutrin on sex drive are, if any, far from instantaneous. In fact, like most antidepressants, Wellbutrin can take weeks or even months to exert its effect. Of course, there is also the consideration of other possible side effects.

Wild yam

Unlike the sweet Thanksgiving Day side dish encrusted with a crunchy brown marshmallow surface, this type of spud isn't nearly as appetizing. The wild yam is an example of yet another poor botanical, ripped from the ground and wrongly credited with being a sex pill.

The abbreviated version on this one seems to follow the false notion that the wild yam contains some sort of hormone that will stimulate one sexually. Unfortunately, all that has been demonstrated is that some species of wild yams contain a substance called "diosgenin." This substance has been shown in laboratory synthesis experiments to produce human sex hormones, but in no way is it by itself a usable human sex hormone. In fact, this in vitro (literally meaning "in glass") laboratory synthesis and conversion of diosgenin to a human sex hormone has never been shown to be possible in vivo (literally meaning "in the human body").

Stemming from the fact that its structure resembles that of the human sex hormones, it does share the same "steroid backbone." But that doesn't make it a human steroid. For example, when we speak of a "steroid" from a chemical standpoint, we are talking about any general structure with three six-carbon rings connected to a five-carbon ring. The simplest of these is cholesterol. When comparing the cholesterol molecule to the testosterone molecule side-by-side, the structural similarity of the steroid backbone in both becomes quite obvious. They are so similar in structure, yet so radically different in function.

What Works and What Doesn't

117

FIGURE 12

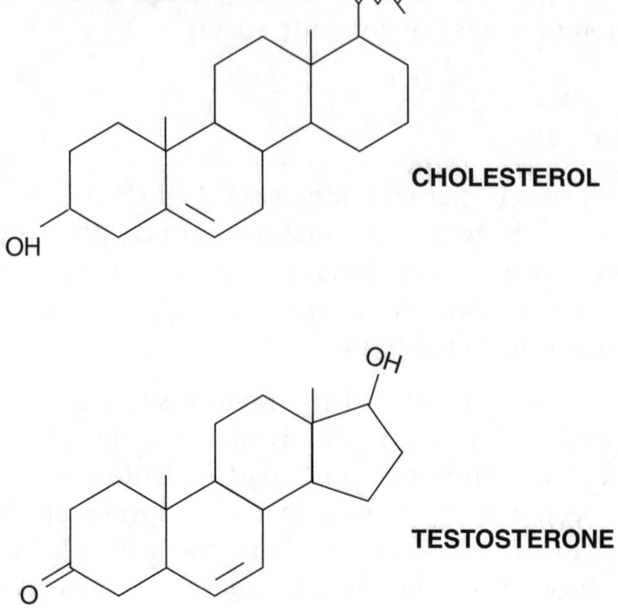

CHOLESTEROL

TESTOSTERONE

= Note the structurally similar steroid backbone in both
molecules outlined in yellow.

Yes, cholesterol is a "steroid." In fact, it is the precursor
to nearly all the steroids found in the human body. These
steroids can be either anabolic (for building up tissue and
substance), catabolic (for breaking down tissue and
combating inflammation), or have a separate function
unrelated to either of these concepts. The most obvious
example of an anabolic steroid is testosterone, while that
of a catabolic steroid is cortisone.

Hence, like humans and animals, plants contain
their own brand of steroid structure compounds. These

compounds are often referred to as "sterols" and are frequently marketed in the bodybuilding world as human steroid substitutes. Herein lies the deception. In the same way cholesterol resembles testosterone in structure, but is radically different in function, so too are the plant sterols. These plant hormones have yet to be demonstrated in legitimate scientific literature as truly usable direct substitutes in humans.

The wild yam is no different, and thus, far from a sex pill. For our purposes, let's turn our attention elsewhere.

Winter Cherry

Derived from the *Withania somnifera* plant in India, the winter cherry is said to be an aphrodisiac. It is believed that when the roots of this potato plant are dried and ground into a fine powder, it can be mixed with milk and drunk before bed to produce a heightened sexual sensitivity. Also known by the Sanskrit name of ashwagandha, the winter cherry is not a total mystery to scientists. In fact, we know this plant contains sleep-inducing alkaloids. In particular, winter cherry contains a small amount of the relatively powerful sleep inducing alkaloid somniferine. When taken in a significant dose, as in the high concentration of the winter cherry root powder, sleep will be all that is induced.

We have a classic case here of science directly contradicting conventional wisdom and ancient folklore. This example serves as a beacon reminder that almost all of the advances in human health and longevity are directly related to our steadfast commitment to traditional medicine. Although alternatives can be effective, decisions to use alternatives should always be tempered with a careful scientific review.

What Works and What Doesn't 119

Yohimbine

Yohimbine is a natural extract derived from the bark of the yohimbe tree that is indigenous to the African Congo. This familiar substance has an interesting mechanism of action and works quite well either by itself or in combination with androstenedione to enhance sexual performance if taken on occasion in a "one-time" dosing fashion. Its action varies considerably for each person taking it, but its variable half-life ranges from about five minutes to almost 8.5 hours in some subjects.

Yohimbine works by temporarily and selectively blocking the sympathetic nervous system. The result is an ability to stave off the male ejaculation, subsequently increasing the duration of intercourse. A male suffering premature ejaculation as a manifestation of sexual dysfunction can hugely benefit from such a natural substance. It differs from substances like Viagra and thus may have a decided advantage for some individuals in terms of effectiveness.

The parasympathic system (aleady mentioned in the context of Viagra) controls arousal, initial erection, and the maintenance of erection. This system controls sexual function throughout the act until the point of ejaculation, at which time the sympathetic system takes over to achieve orgasm.

Yohimbine works by locally blocking the sympathetic nerve system. Recall that this system is "counter" to the parasympathetic system that dominates throughout erection. As mentioned, the sympathetic system activates and takes over at the point of ejaculation. This is achieved via an "adrenergic" chemical neurotransmitter-based stimulation of what is called the "alpha-2" receptor. Yohimbine, which is a selective alpha-2 blocker can effectively impede this stimulation. Simply put, the theory is that yohimbine can temporarily block the sympathetic nerve stimulation that governs orgasm and thus stave off the male ejaculation, subsequently increasing the duration of intercourse.

"Mechanism of Action of Yohimbine:"

1. Parasympathetic Nerve Stimulation;

↓

2. **Arousal Phase** (erection via nitric oxide-cGMP mechanism in Figure 1);

↓

3. **Excitation Phase** (maintenance of erection throughout intercourse is governed by continued parasympathetic stimulation);

↓

YOHIMBINE (alpha-2 blockade) ⟶ ▬

↓

4. **Ejaculation** (a rapid switch over to the sympathetic system and subsequent stimulation of the alpha-2 receptor results in the male orgasm and termination of erection);

↓

5. **Recfractory Phase** (the phase at which time sympathetic stimulation continues to dominate and further stimulation will not result in erection);

↓

6. **Recovery Phase** (both parasympathetic and sympathetic systems are iin balance again and arousal by parasympathetic stimulation can again be achieved).

Yohimbine can be taken alone both in prescription and over-the-counter forms. Unfortunately, given its mechanism of action, it will really only stave off ejaculation, for the most part. However, theoretically one might draw the conclusion that by blocking sympathetic stimulation you might enhance the pure effectiveness of parasympathetic stimulation. Again in theory, during the arousal and excitation phases the idea that the counter force of sympathetic input can be blocked, the parasympathetic input is free to govern erection and enhance these phases as well. Unfortunately, "theory" and "clinical practice" are two very different things. My colleagues in the field inform me that yohimbine does not seem to effectively enhance these earlier phases. (For the purpose of enhancing these phases, substances like Viagra and pure androstenedione clearly win out over yohimbine alone). It's enough to say that if premature ejaculation is your issue, great. But if libido enhancing is also a concern, the preference would clearly be toward a combination of yohimbine extract and androstenedione.

Remember, when selecting a sex pill, you need to identify the area you want to improve. By this I mean specifically, is your libido adequate but your performance poor (i.e., pre-mature ejaculation)? Is your problem solely an issue of libido (i.e., flattened sexual desire)? Maybe both aspects are suffering. Of course there are also those vigorous gentlemen in which plumbing and psyche are working fine, but these studs simply want too much of a good thing in both areas (careful—not a safe mind-set).

Yohimbine, taken by itself, is not without its downside. Something to consider when using yohimbine alone as a sexual enhancer is the element of anxiety. No well-read scientist would challenge the effectiveness of yohimbine. But when taken in excess, it can result in extreme nervousness and anxiety. This is something that is sure to snub sexual desire and end up doing the exact opposite of what you wanted it for in the first place. So, although yohimbine is quite a reasonable option as a sex pill, you must be extremely careful not to overdose and get the reverse effect—a classic case of more not being better! A safer bet is to combine yohimbine with other natural sex pills. As mentioned, perhaps the best single natural, non-prescription sex pill combination is androstenedione with yohimbine as found in TWINLAB's AndroFuel™. By combining these unique and highly effective substances, the individual dosage requirement is minimized while the added benefit of potent complimentary synergy is achieved.

Zinc

Zinc is a mineral nutrient essential to innumerable chemical pathways in the human body including its role in the molecular structure of at least 100 different enzymes. We know that zinc functions as an antioxidant, promoting growth, development and wound healing. Although available in fairly significant levels in lean red meat, chicken hearts, lamb, fish, and eggs, zinc supplementation comes in the form of vitamin tablets either in pure form or, more commonly, mixed in with a multivitamin complex.

Because zinc is essential in the normal growth, differentiation and maintenance of the male reproductive system, it has incorrectly been labeled as a sexual enhancer by some. This mislabeling may well stem from the fact that zinc deficiency has been associated with delayed sexual maturity in children and low hormone production in adults.

Although many men over the age of 40 have measurable zinc deficiency and are effectively supplemented with exogenous zinc, this generally does not translate to sexual enhancement. Of course, in cases of profound and overt zinc deficiency, sexual function will likely be depressed. When this particular derangement in bodily zinc titer is corrected, it may appear as if zinc exerted some kind of direct action on correcting sexual function. Unfortunately, under conditions of normal physiology and nutrition, the idea of excess zinc as an enhancer of sexual activity could not be further from the truth.

CONCLUSION

Amid this plethora of sex pills, one can't help but sit back in wonderment and amazement at the magnitude of the list. Bear in mind that this list is in no way comprehensive. The fact is, there are innumerable pills, cocktails, potions, elixirs, and creams that have been labeled either accurately or inaccurately with sex-enhancing powers. Crossing cultures, spanning world geography, and even tribal and religious rituals, the notion of the sex pill is nothing short of commonplace. At base, sex is the primary life purpose and the primordial pleasure that universally drives us all. Thus, the global fixation on a substance that can stimulate or further enhance this euphoric primal act should come as no surprise.

Keep in mind that this text is in no way a finite retrospective. Rather, as the general human need to enhance the sexual act cannot be squelched by either time or the constraints of religious or politically motivated beliefs, the list must keep growing.

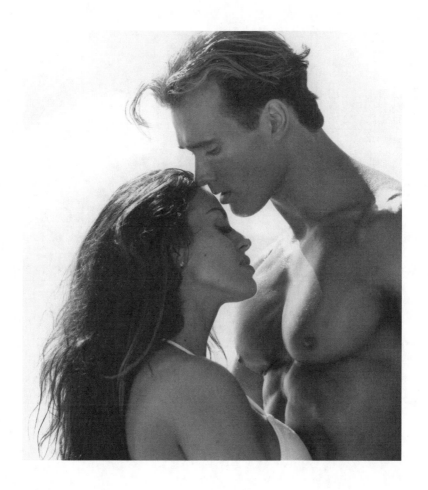

Sex Pills

SELECTED REFERENCES

1. Aldercreutz H (1990). Western diet and western diseases: Some hormonal and biochemical mechanisms and associations. Scand. J. Clin. Lab. Invest. 50(20):3-20.

2. Aldercreutz H (1991). Diet and sex hormone metabolism. In Nutrition, Toxicity, and Cancer. (Edited by I.R. Rowland). CRC Press, Boca Raton. pp. 137-195.

3. Anon., Ginseng: Western myth or Easern promise? IPU Rev1 994;69(9).

4. Adlercreutz H, Bannwart C, Wahala K (1993). Inhibition of human aromatase by mammalian lignans and isoflavonoid phytoestrogens. J. Steroid Biochem. Molec. Biol. 44(2): 147-153.

5. American Heart Association; FDA: Medical Tribune (www.medtrib.com/fp8.htm).

6. Berges R, Windeler J, Trampisch H (1995). Randomized, placebo-controlled, double blind clinical trial of beta-sistosterol in patients with benign prostatic hyperplasia. Lancet. 345:1529.

7. Barret-Conner, E, (1986). A prospective study of DHEAS, mortality and cardiovascular disease. N. Engl. J. Med.; 315(24):1519-1524.

8. Betz J, White K (1995). Gas chromatographic determination of yohimbine in commercial yohimbine products. J. AOAC Int. 78(5):1189-1194.

9. Beinfeld, H., Between Heaven and Earth: A Guide to Chinese Medicine. New York. Ballatine Books, 1991.

10. Block, G., et al. Fruit, vegetables, and cancer prevention: A review of the epidemiological evidence. Nutr. Cancer 18:1-29, 1992.

11. Bradlow H (1998). Indole-3-carbinole and estrogen metabolism: A biochemical approach to cancer chemoprevention. International Conference on Cancer Prevention. Strang Cancer Center, New York, NY.

What Works and What Doesn't

12. Brodie A (1991). Aromatase and its inhibitors—an overview. J. Steroid Biochem. Molec. Biol.. 40(1-3): 255

13. Burnett A (1992). Nitric Oxide: A physiologic mediator of penile erection. Science. July 17; .257:401.

14. Casson PR, (1997). DHEA replacement after menopause? Too early to tell. Patient Care. 31(11):147-155.

15. Crane B, Avrai A, Dipak G (1998). Structure of nitric oxide synthase oxygenase dimer with pterin and substrate. Science. March 27; 279:2121-2126.

16. Cross-gender sex pill. Time. April 6, 1998.

17. Curci A, Pjevi, Radeka G (1996). [Nutritional status in women and estrogen production in surgical menopause]. Medicinski fakultet 49:1-2, 54-56.

18. Daviies JH, Dowsett M, Jacobs S (1992). Aromatase inhibition: 4-hydroxyandrostenedione in advanced prostatic cancer. Br. J. Cancer. 66(1): 139-42.

19. Demling L (1991). Urological and sexual evaluation of treatment of benign prostatic disease using Pygeum africanum at high dose. Arch. Ital. Urol. Nefrol. Androl. 63:341-345.

20. Disilverio F, D'Eramo G, Lubrano C (1992). Evidence that *Serenoa repens* extract displays an antiestrogenic activity in prostatic tissue of benign prostatic hypertrophy patients. Eur. Urol. 21:309-314.

21. Duke JA, (1995). Handbook of Medicinal Herbs. Boca Raton: CRC Press.

22. Ernst E, pittler MH (1998). Yohimbine for erectile dysfunction. A systemic review and meta-analysis of randomized clinical trials. J. Urol. 159:433-436.

23. Farnsworth N (1985). *Eleutherococcus sennticosus:* current status as an adaptogen. Econ. Med. Plant Res. 1:156-215.

24. FDC Reports 1998; "The Pink Sheet". 60;(13):3.

25. Feenstra J (1998). Acute myocardial infarction associated with sildenafil. The Lancet. 352:957.

26. Felter H (1983). The Eclectic Materia Medica, Pharmacology and Therapeutics. Portland, OR: Eclectic Medical Publications.

27. First pill to treat erectile dysfunction approved. Medical Tribune: Internist & Cardiologist Edition. April 16, 1998.

28. Harrison's 12th Ed. Principles of Internal Medicine. Vol. 1& 2. 1997 McGraw-Hill. New York, NY.

29. Fontenot B (1998). The hyping of DHEA: long on claims, short on evidence. Nutrition Forum; 15(1):3-7.

30. Foster, Steven. Ginkgo Biloba: A living fossil for today's health needs. Better Nutrition, November 1996, V. 58, No. 11.

31. Fox News-Colorado (1998). Channel 31: television interview with Andrew Weil, M.D. January 5.

32. Goldberg B (1997). Alternative Medicine, The Definitive Guide. Puyallup, Washington: The Burton Goldberg Group.

33. Gottlieb B (1995). New Choices in Natural Healing. Rodale Press.

34. Griffith H (1988). Complete Guide to Vitamins, Minerals, and Supplements. Fisher Books. Tucson, Arizona.

35. Groff, James, et al (1998). Advanced nutrition and human metabolism. Second Edition.

36. Harrison's 12th Ed. (1997). Principles of Internal Medicine. Vol. 1& 2.

37. Health Library. www.thriveonline.com.

38. Hoffken K, Jonat W, Possinger K (1991). Aromatase inhibition with 4-hydroxyadrostenedione in the treatment of postmenopausal patients with advanced breast cancer: A phase II study. J. Clinical Oncology. 8(5): 875-80.

39. Ibrahim AR, Abul-Hajj YJ (1990). Aromatase inhibition by flavonoids. J. Steroid Biochem. Molec. Biol. 37(2): 257-260.

40. Johan's Guide to Aphrodisiacs. www.santesson.com.

41. Katzung BG. Editor (1989) Basic and clinical pharmacology. Fourth edition. Appleton and Lange. Norwalk, CT.

42. Kellis JT, Vickery LE (1984). Inhibition of human estrogen synthetase (aromatase) by flavones. Science. 225: 1032-34.

43. Kindersley, Dorling. (1997) The complete medicinal herbal handbook: A practical guide to the healing properties of herbs with more than 250 remedies for common ailments. London, England and New York, NY.

44. Lamm S, (1998). The virility solution. Simon and Schuster.

45. Mahesh and R.B. Greenblatt (1962). The in vivo conversion of dehydroepiandrosterone and androstenedione to testosterone in the human. Acta Endo-crinol. 41:400-406.

46. Mechcatie E, (1995). Can testosterone treat more than just libido? Internal Medicine News. July 1. p16.

47. Merz PG, (1996). The effects of a special agnus cactus extract (BP1095E1) on prolactin secretion in healthy male subjects. Exp Clin Endocrin Diab 104:447-53.

48. Murray M (1998). Encyclopedia of natural medicine. 2nd Edition. Rocklin, California: Prima Publishing.

49. National Research Council (1989). Recommended Dietary Allowances 10th Ed., National Academy Press, pp. 52-77.

50. Pierpoint W.S. (1986). Flavonoids in the human diet. In Plant Flavonoids in Biology and Medicine. (Edited by V. Cody, E. Middleton and J. Harborne). Liss, New York. Pp. 125-140.

51. Pfizer's impotence pill receives FDA approval. The New York Times. March 30, 1998.

52. Schnirring L, (198). DHEA: Hype, hope not matched by facts. The Phys. Sportsmed. Vol26, No. 5, pp. 17-22.

53. Schumm D, (1997). Essentials of Biochemistry. Little, Brown and Company, Massachusetts, pp. 334-340.

54. Sex Pill of the 90's. www.doctorg.com.

55. Shackleton C, Roitman E, Phillips A, Chang T (1997). Androstenediol and 5-androstenediol profiling for detecting exogenously administered dihydrotestosterone, epitestosterone, and dehydroepiandrosterone: Potential use in gas chromatography isotope ratio mass spectrometry. Steroids. 62:665-673.

56. Sherman, Carl. Some herbal remedies may be useful anxiolytics. Internal Medicine News. June 15, 1998.

57. Singleton V.L. (1981). Naturally occurring food toxicants: Phenolic substances of plant origin common in foods. Adv.Food Res. 27: 149-242.

58. Skolnick A (1996), Scientific verdict still out on DHEA. JAMA; 276(17): 1365-1367.

59. Sturgill, Marc G., et al (1997). Yohimbine elimination in normal volunteers is characterized by both one- and two-compartment behavior. J. Cardiov. Pharm. 29: 697-703.

60. The new impotence drug. USA Today. March 31, 1998.

61. Ueda S, Petrie J, Cleland S (1998). Insulin vasodilatation and the "arginine paradox". The Lancet. 351:959-960.

62. U.S. approves sale of impotence pill. The New York Times. March 28, 1998.

63. Vitali G (1995). Carnitine supplementation in human idiopathic asthenospermia: Clinical results. Drugs Exp. Clin. Res. 21:157-159.

64. Wierman M, Cassel C (1998). Erectile dysfunction: a multifaceted disorder. Hospital Practice. October 15, 1998. 65-90.

65. Zorgniotti A, Lizza E (1994). Effect of large doses of the nitric oxide precursor, L-arginine, on erectile dysfunction. Int. J. Impotence Res. 6:33-36.

GLOSSARY

amino acid – Considered "the building blocks of protein," amino acids play a vital role in the production and regulation of brain chemicals.

amphetamine - A drug that stimulates the central nervous system, it is often used to lift mood in cases of depression or control appetite in cases of obesity.

anabolic – Relating to the conversion of simple to more complex nutritive material to promote muscle and tissue growth; constructive metabolism.

androgenic – Any substance, natural or synthetic, that promotes masculine characteristics. Testosterone is an androgen.

andropausal – Adaptation of the word menopausal, but as it might be applied to males rather than females; "male menopause."

androstendione – An androgenic steroid that can be converted metabolically to testosterone and other androgens.

aphrodisiac – A chemical agent, food, drug, potion or odor that stimulates sexual desire.

aromatase inhibitor – A molecule or agent that prevents the enzymatic coversion of androgens to estrogens.

atropine – A poisonous substance from belladonna and other plants of the nightshade family that prevents the response of various body structures to certain types of nerve stimulation.

cancer – A malignant tumor that arises from the abnormal and uncontrolled division of cells that destroy surrounding tissue.

chronic – Marked by long duration or frequent recurrence, as in many medical conditions.

DDT – A colorless, odorless, water-insoluble insecticide found to have a toxic affect on many vertebrates. Its agricultural use has been banned in the U.S. since 1973.

Sex Pills

DHEA – A steroid hormone (dehydroepiandrosterone) naturally produced in the adrenal glands that is also sold in synthetic form as a nutritional supplement.

dilate – To make wider or larger; to cause to expand.

endogenous – Developing from within the body.

edema – accumulation of fluid in tissue cells that results in swelling.

endocrinology – The branch of biology dealing with the endocrine glands and their hormonal secretions. The endocrines include the pituitary, thyroid, parathyroid and adrenal glands, the ovary and testis, the placenta, and part of the pancreas.

enzymatic – Pertaining to various proteins capable of producing chemical changes in organic substances without being consumed in the process.

ergogenic – The quality of being able to enhance work capacity or performance.

estrogen – Any of a group of major female sex hormones that stimulate the development of female secondary sex characteristics.

estrogen therapy – Estrogen supplementation, often called ERT (estrogen replacement therapy) given to some menopausal and post-menopausal women to reduce the risk of osteoporosis and other health problems caused by lowered natural estrogen levels.

flavone – A colorless, water-insoluble compound found in the leaves, stems and seed capsules of many primroses; any of the derivatives of this compound that occur as yellow plant pigments and are used as dyes.

free radicals – Molecules in the body that have one or more unpaired electrons and are extremely reactive, tending to destabilize other molecules causing tissue damage. Some of the more destructive free radicals derive from oxygen.

gynecomastia – Abnormal enlargement of the breast in a male.

half life – The time required for half the amount of a substance or drug introduced into a living organism to be eliminated or disintegrated by natural processes.

hallucinogenic – Pertaining to hallucinations, which are sensory experiences of something that does not exist outside the mind. They can be caused by various physical or mental disorders or by reaction to toxic substances.

hypogonadism – Diminished hormonal or reproductive functioning in the testes or ovaries that retards sexual development.

hysterectomy – Surgical removal of the uterus.

insulin – A protein hormone produced by the pancreas that regulates the metabolism of glucose and other nutrients. It is used in the treatment and control of diabetes mellitus.

interstitial cells – The cells interspersed between the tubules of the testis. They secrete androgens in response to stimulation by luteinizing hormone from the pituitary gland; Leydig cells.

isoflavone – A naturally occurring plant component that shares similarities with estrogen.

luteinizing hormone – A hormone synthesized and released by the pituitary gland that stimulates ovulation, progesterone synthesis by the ovary, and androgen synthesis by the interstitial cells of the testes.

libido – The emotional energy derived from primitive biological urges; sex drive.

lymphocyte – A type of white blood present in the lymph nodes, spleen, thymus, gut wall and bone marrow. They are involved in immunity.

menopause – The period of permanent cessation of menstruation that usually occurs between the ages of 45 and 55.

menstrual disturbances – Problems surrounding the monthly discharge of blood and mucosal tissue from the uterus.

metastatic disease – The spread of disease-producing organisms or of cancerous cells from the organ or tissue of origin to another part of the body.

Sex Pills

naturopathic – Pertaining to a system of treating disease that employs no surgery or synthetic drugs, but instead uses special diets, herbs, vitamins, massage, etc. to assist natural healing processes.

neuro-hormonal pathway – The delivery system of blood vessels through which hormonal substances formed in the nervous system flow to appropriate organs of the body.

non-essentail amino acid – Amino acids that can be synthesized by the body. By contrast, essential amino acids must be obtained from protein in the diet.

PCBs – Polychlorinated biphenyls; a family of highly toxic organic compounds that persist in the environment. They are known to cause skin diseases and are suspected of causing birth defects and cancer.

pharmacokinetic metabolism – The manner in which the body uses various pharmacological substances.

phytoestrogen – An estrogen-like compound derived from plants.

placebo – A substance having no pharmacological effect that is given as a control in testing experimentally or clinically the efficacy of another substance.

postmenopausal – Relating to the period in a woman's life following the complete cessation of menstruation.

primary hypogonadism – See hypogonadism.

prolactin – A pituitary hormone that stimulates lactation by the mammary glands after childbirth and also stimulates production of progesterone in the ovary.

prostate – An organ that surrounds the urethra in males at the base of the bladder. It comprises a muscular portion that controls the release of urine and a glandular portion that secretes an alkaline fluid that makes up part of the semen.

psychoactive – Pertaining to a substance having a profound effect on mental processes.

radical prostatectomy – Surgical removal of the entire prostate gland.

scopolomine – A water-soluble alkaloid obtained from certain plants of the nightshade family and used as a sedative, to prevent muscle spasm, and to relieve the symptoms of motion sickness.

sexual dysfunction – Disturbance, impairment or abnormality in the functioning of the genital organs.

sphincter – A specialized ring of muscle that surrounds an opening through which something may pass.

steroid – Any of a large group of fat-soluble organic compounds, such as the sex hormones or bile acids, most of which have specific physiological action.

sublingual – Situated under the tongue or on the underside of the tongue.

suppository – A solid form of a medicinal preparation that melts upon insertion into the rectum or vagina.

testosterone – The principal male sex hormone. It is secreted by the testes and stimulates development of the male sex organs, secondary sexual traits and sperm.

thrombophlebitis – The presence of a thrombus (fibrinous blood clot) in a vein accompanied by inflammation of the vessel wall.

transdermal – Able to be applied to the skin, usually as part of an adhesive patch, for absorption into the bloodstream.

Appendix A

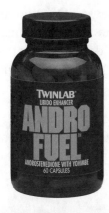

One (1) ANDRO FUEL® capsule provides:

Androstenedione..........................100 mg
   (Pure Pharmaceutical Grade)

Yohimbe Bark Extract ....400 mg
   (Standardized for 8 mg yohimbine)

RECOMMENDED USE: As a dietary supplement for men, take 1-2 capsules sixty minutes before sex. Do not exceed two capsules daily, 1-3 times weekly.

TWINLAB® ANDRO FUEL®
IS AVAILABLE FROM THE FOLLOWING COMPANIES

TWINLAB®
150 Motor Parkway
Hauppauge, NY 11788

Available at Fine Retail Stores Everywhere

BRONSON®
600 East Quality Drive
American Fork, UT 84003

Order Direct 24 hours a day, 7 days a week
Telephone: 1-800-235-3200
Fax: 1-801-756-5739

ADVANCED RESEARCH PRESS PUBLICATIONS

(To Order Call 1-888-841-8007 *Except Where Noted)

The Cooking Cardiologist *(Video - 50 Minutes)* - Dr. Richard Collins, a cardiologist and leading researcher on reversing heart disease discusses and demonstrates how to cook delicious healthy meals that can lessen the risk of cardiovascular disease and improve one's overall health - 50 minute video. $19.95

The Cooking Cardiologist by Dr. Richard Collins - over 350 luscious recipes to lower cholesterol reduce the risk of heart disease, lower weight and improve health through the addition of plant proteins, fiber, and foods high in 3-omega fatty acids to your favorite recipes. Hard cover, 224 pages. $21.95

The Consumer's Guide To Herbal Medicine by Dr. Steven B. Karch, M.D. - a professional medical review of 65 of the most widely used herbs, their use, benefits and effectiveness; safety considerations, drug interactions, including German Government Commission E recommendations of which every user of herbs should be aware. Hard cover, 224 pages. $29.95

Tomato Power by James F. Scheer with Forward by James F. Balch, M.D. - discusses the benefits of a super-antioxidant, lycopene, that can slow aging and reduce heart disease and cancer risks. Soft cover, 144 pages. $12.95

Sex Pills A-Z, from Androstenedione to Zinc. *What Works and What doesn't!* by Dr. Carlon M. Colker, M.D. - examines a plethora of sex enhancing substances for added pleasure, better sex, longer sex, restoring sex drive, reversing sexual dysfunction and improving sexual powers. Soft cover, 128 pages. $14.95

Optimum Sports Nutrition, *Your Competitive Edge,* by Dr. Michael Colgan - a complete guide to the nutritional requirements of athletes. Soft cover, 562 pages. $24.95

Muscular Development magazine - brings its readers the very best and latest scientific information on strength training, physique development, nutrition, health and fitness in an entertaining and contemporary format. 12 issues, ($2.50/copy - 50% off cover price). $29.94

Living Longer In The Boomer Age by Dr. John L. Zenk M.D. - discusses integrating alternative and conventional medicine. He describes the benefits of a new miracle anti-aging miracle supplement, 7-Keto DHEA for improving the immune system, losing fat and enhancing memory. *To order call 1-888-841-7996. $9.95

Periodization Breakthrough! *The Ultimate Training System* by Drs. Fleck and Kraemer. A straightforward explanation of periodized training. An essential system for successful strength training. Hard cover, 182 pages *To order call 1-888-841-7996. $19.95

Muscle Meals by John Romano - a cookbook for bodybuilders and all athletes featuring a delicious array of easy-to-prepare energy-packed low-fat meals. Written by culinary expert, TV chef on ESPN's American Muscle Meals. Hard cover, 224 pages. *To order call 1-888-841-7996. $19.95

Mike Mentzer (New Advanced) High Intensity Training Program - a series of 4 audio-taped lectures, each approximately 50 minutes, by Mike Mentzer, Mr. Universe Champion, student and master of the art of bodybuilding. Included with these tapes is a 40 page High Intensity Training Program Guide; all attractively packaged. *To order call 1-888-841-7996. $39.95

INTERNET ORDERS

*These items can also be ordered via the internet
www.advancedresearchpress.com
click on the product mall to view.